Melanie Verwoerd is a former
Parliament, South African Amba:
Director of UNICEF Ireland. Sh
presenter, columnist and top-rated political analyst from Cape
Town, South Africa.

Melanie grew up during the height of Apartheid in South Africa.
At the age of twenty she married Wilhelm Verwoerd, the
grandson of the former Apartheid Prime Minister HF Verwoerd,
generally regarded as the architect of Apartheid. In 1990, after
a brief spell at Oxford in the UK and following the unbanning of
the ANC, she and her then husband returned to South Africa.

Shortly after their return Melanie met with Nelson Mandela,
who encouraged her to "use her surname and voice for the
bigger good". She stunned many by joining the ANC. Her
involvement led to her being ostracized by her community and
numerous death threats. During the first democratic elections
in 1994 - at the age of 27 - Melanie became the youngest female
MP ever to be elected in South Africa. She was re-elected in
1999 and in 2001 was appointed as South African Ambassador
to Ireland. In 2007 she became head of UNICEF Ireland. She
returned to Cape Town in 2013.

Also by Melanie Verwoerd:

When We Dance
The Verwoerd that Toyi-Toyied
*Our Madiba: stories and reflections from those who met Nelson
Mandela*
21@21: The coming of age of a nation.

Praise

The women and men below are not A-listers or book reviewers. They are the ones I wrote this book for. People like you and me.

Dr. Erika Mitchell MD (South Africa): I devoured this book while internalising the humorous, beautifully poised words and gentle wisdom. The looping storyline; clever chronology; heartfelt originality and clarity of thinking are a gem. Wow! Truly, the work of an artist and a creator.

I felt a little as I did when I finished Glennon Doyle's *Untamed* - inspired, open, heart-touched, slightly in love with the author.

******

Katie Trippe (USA): Wow! I didn't want to put this book down…. It's like sipping a warm tea, comforting and funny and relatable and raw. I LOVED IT!

******

Dr. Luz Longworth Phd (Jamaica): In this book Melanie succeeds not only in finding her voice again but voicing a plethora of emotions that women are often unable or unwilling to express their own loss, love and triumph. I enjoyed it, suffered with Melanie through it and emerged triumphant and positive with her at the end. Thank you, Melanie, for your courage in revealing yourself to us so that we may be brave enough to embark on our own journey to ourselves.

******

Rita-Marie Hopfner (Australia): A deeply introspective journey into what we associate with our feminine selves and what we believe defines us as women. I felt every raw emotion in this must-read story about one woman's experience of hysterectomy.

******

Denise Dixon (Antiqua): Real. Raw. Riveting. Any woman who has faced a traumatic, life altering experience (and we've all had at least one) knows the pain, the grief, the anger that come with personal crisis. All the feelings we find creative ways to cover up, Melanie unpacks as she tells her story. This book was a lifeline for me. I laughed, I cried and most of all, I left feeling inspired to continue on my own journey of healing.

******

Abraham le Roux (South Africa): As a Clinical Psychologist, I recommend Melanie's book as a must read for any woman and her partner that is suddenly confronted with a life changing reality. Her kind, sound and thorough approach, will be a great support.

******

Malcolm Nicholls (New Zealand): This book is a must read for men (and women) whose partners are going through a crisis. Having supported my wife through her cancer journey I know it can be terribly confusing and scary not knowing or understanding what the hell is happening. Read this book for yourself and your partner. It could change everything....

******

Jo Lennert (South Africa): Melanie is a true storyteller. The way her experience is intertwined with historical events makes it even more enjoyable. Women truly need to share knowledge and support each other as she does in this book.

******

Nadine McNeil (Jamaica): This book is a must read, especially for persons who dare to take a deep, inside look at what it truly means to be a woman. It is only through these harrowing experiences that we often learn about ourselves and our bodies. Despite having endured this ordeal -- one that I can comfortably say all menopausal women especially secretly dread -- Melanie's story is one of grace, vulnerability and triumph. Through her sharing, the reader gets an 'up close and personal' view of ALL the aspects that are involved in this life-altering process. As she takes us deep into the vestiges of her life experiences, we realize that just like her we too can and will overcome and continue to thrive in this new and largely unfamiliar terrain of life.

******

Reverend Prof. Peter Storey (South Africa): A warm, brave and nakedly honest book for women that every man should read.

******

Brid Walls (Ireland): Absolutely amazing! I couldn't put it down.

******

Never Waste a Good Hysterectomy
Life lessons from a crisis

Melanie Verwoerd

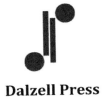

Dalzell Press

First published in 2023 by Dalzell Press

Dalzell Press
54 Abbey Street
Bangor, N. Ireland
BT20 4JB

ISBN 978-1-8380871-6-6

To the millions of women around the world whose stories will never be told.

May you wear your scars with pride.

"Write the tale that scares you,
That makes you feel uncertain,
That isn't comfortable.
I dare you..."

Michaela Cole

Foreword

Courage...

Brené Brown says that "courage" is a heart word.

I like that.

She also says that in its earliest form the word meant "to speak one's mind by telling all one's heart."

The mere idea of that scares the living daylights out of me. I'm a deeply private person and despite – or perhaps because of – having been in the public eye all of my adult life, I don't like people knowing my business, particularly those bits we usually don't speak about.

Still, I had no choice.

This had to be a book full of heart words.

It is a book of heartfulness.

A friend once reminded me that we only ever write for ourselves. We write to heal and all we can hope for is that we might help others in the process.

I wrote this book primarily to come to terms with what happened to me.

That required me to lay myself bare – something that demanded enormous courage. Some might find uncomfortable to read, but I know that there are countless women around the world who will identify with what I went through, but will never have their stories heard.

This book is meant for them.

May my words vibrate in your heart and may they help you to find the courage to deal with whatever you are facing in your life.

And: Let us hold hands together and tell our stories – with all our heart, because they deserve to be heard!

Diving into the pain

"How are you?" asked George, my vet.

"Better, thanks," I replied whilst giving my Golden Retriever the evil eye.

Two-year old Blue was lying half asleep on the floor. Every now and then, he suffers from postnasal drip and thinks he's got something stuck in his throat. (What he lacks in intelligence he makes up for in cuteness.) This would send him into a frenzy, running around, barking loudly to be let outside. Once in the garden he would eat grass at a rate that would impress the biggest Jersey cow. Sometimes it would help, but mostly we would end up at the vet to get a steroid injection (him, not me). I'm not sure George believes the whole gulping, grass-eating panic, since it disappears miraculously every time we arrive at his surgery.

It had been one of those days.

After two frantic hours of barking and grass eating, I got an emergency appointment. Gulping and gasping all the way to the vet, Blue made an instantaneous recovery the moment we arrived. He ran into the practice, greeted the receptionists who confirmed that he was still gorgeous and then sat down on the scale without being prompted. When George (and his tin of biscuits) arrived he nearly died of excitement. The injection took five seconds, the biscuit one second and now he was snoring loudly on the surgery floor, which was when George turned to me.

"I'm not only talking about the physical trauma," he said. "After what you've gone through there must be enormous emotional trauma as well."

For a moment I wondered if it was his way of saying: "It's not the dog that has a problem...", but I then saw the empathy in his eyes and I welled up unexpectedly.

While I fought back tears, I reflected on the irony that a man who on a daily basis performs hysterectomies on dogs and cats was the one who validated what I had been feeling for weeks.

THIS HAD BEEN A FUCKING BIG DEAL AND I WAS NOT FINE!!

That night I was lying in bed unable to sleep. My heart was racing and my body felt wound up as anxious thoughts sped around my brain.

I was exhausted yet couldn't sleep. "Why was I so tired?" I wondered. I hadn't done anything for the past eight weeks.

Perhaps that was exactly it. After all, the physical recovery was damn hard work. It certainly had been no holiday – and a holiday is what I now craved.

I wanted to get time to be still, to be able to make sense of what had happened to me since the fateful visit to the gynaecologist ten weeks earlier.

Instead, the eight weeks of sick leave was running out in a few days, and I had to get back to work.

Work?

The thought of having to follow the daily temper tantrums of South African politicians made me groan out loud. It seemed so mundane in the light of what had happened to me.

"I think I have a form of PTSD."

The thought was demanding attention.

I rolled it around in my brain.

I had been so busy dealing with the all-absorbing demands of physical recovery, I had ignored the emotional trauma. It wasn't that I didn't realise it was there – I had just thought that recognising its existence would be enough.

I should have known better. After all, it was not my first rodeo. A decade before, I was thrown into a hurricane of trauma and grief after my partner died. It took years of hard work to regain my balance.

So here I was again....

From my earlier work with psychologists and trauma councillors, I knew that talking helped. The more we relive the trauma the less emotionally charged the event becomes and the weaker the psychological impact.

Was that why I was now telling everyone willing – and not so willing – about what happened? I even wrote a piece about it for a big online newspaper. How much of it was awareness-raising and how much was my brain and body remembering the lessons of ten years ago?

Staring at the ceiling, I knew that the reasons didn't really matter. All I knew was that it helped.

Words help.

In my mind I heard Maya Angelou's deep voice: "Words are things – powerful things. So be careful how you use them."

I put the light on and grabbed my laptop. I started to type frantically. This was my way of eating grass.

Of making sense.

Of trying to breathe again.

Of looking forward.

I was no longer the same person.

After a big trauma no one ever is.

When the shock comes your DNA gets rewired and you are no longer the same.

I was a different person.

Physically, I had less organs and more scars. Emotionally, I was bruised and battered.

I knew I had no choice.

To quote P!nk, I had to dive deep into the pain of the last few weeks. I had to wrap my brain around what happened, in order to welcome the change it must bring.

After all, it would be a terrible waste of a good hysterectomy if life was to go on as before.

When dam walls collapse

"What's going on here?"

My usually chatty gynaecologist had suddenly gone quiet and was leaning closer to the ultrasound screen. I watched her face as she zoomed into the images.

"Do you have any pain?" she asked. "No, nothing!" I said firmly, thinking that it would negate whatever she was seeing on the shadowy images of my organs. From the way her frown deepened it was clearly not the answer she was hoping for.

A feeling of foreboding started to vibrate deep in my stomach – the second time today.

"I'm going for my regular gynae visit," I had told my daughter earlier. "Say hallo!" she said cheerfully, since we shared the same gynaecologist. Thinking about the upcoming visit, I was suddenly overwhelmed by a sense of dread. It surprised me. I don't mind going to the gynaecologist. I have been making these annual visits like a faithful pilgrim since I was 17 – which means at least 37 visits. Added to that a number of extra pap smears when I got abnormal test results for a few years, the removal of two Bartholin's cysts and the births of my two children – hell, my vagina was almost public property.

I had pushed the negative thoughts aside, putting it down to a lack of social engagement during COVID, but lying with my legs in stirrups while the gynaecologist was moving the probe around, it felt like I was standing next to a high dam wall watching big cracks forming.

"I need you to go up to the pathologists for a CA125 test," the gynaecologist said. "Now?" I asked.

"Yes." A weird kindness had crept into her voice.

"What are we testing for?" I asked.

"Cancer," she replied.

The dam wall started to crumble.

"A CA 125 test may be used to look for early signs of ovarian cancer," I read on my phone as I waited for the lift to arrive. The article went on to describe the five-year survival rates for ovarian cancer. It was shocking.

"I won't have cancer," I tried to console myself. "I am too healthy".

However, by the time the lift doors had opened two floors up, my world had changed. The article I was planning to write seemed trite, I couldn't care less about my clients' anxieties, about the current political drama, and the domestic chores I had on my lists were forgotten.

"I might have cancer," was all I could think.

I recognised the phlebotomist from a cholesterol test ten months before. We talked about her having had COVID a second time since I had seen her last. "How are you?" she asked. I felt tears welling up.

"I'm a bit freaked out to be honest."

She glanced over at the form with the codes for the various tests. I saw her eyes widening slightly. "Try not to worry too much. It might be nothing," she said with the same weird tone of kindness in her voice.

The next day the results were back. The tumour markers were elevated.

"Don't start planning your funeral yet," a medical cousin said, "it could just be a cyst, but they will have to do more tests".

While listening to him, I thought of the story of the little boy trying to stop the dam wall from collapsing with his finger.

The gynaecologist called two days later to say that she had spoken to a gynaecological oncologist. He was going on holiday but would see me in two weeks. She also mentioned that he was certain that a hysterectomy would be necessary.

My head started to spin. "Why an oncologist? Surely they don't know that I have cancer. Or do they? Surgery? Hysterectomy? I have to wait for two weeks to know more?"

Through my anxiety I felt an anger rising. This man (!) had

already decided to do a hysterectomy without even having seen me or doing further tests. Surely there should be a few steps before just cutting into me and removing... I wasn't even sure what they would remove.

I felt like I was on a roller coaster picking up speed – it was terrifying and there was no way of getting off.

I needed to think, to regain a sense of control.

That night I called one of my best friends in Ireland. Elaine is one of the most compassionate and brilliant GPs I have ever met. She is a genius and I have literally trusted her with my life since we met 20 years ago. "In Ireland we would definitely do more tests. At a minimum a CT scan," she said. "Also, that blood test is not very reliable to diagnose ovarian cancer if you haven't had it before, plus your tumour markers are only slightly elevated. Cancer is usually above 300." (Normally the markers should be below 35, mine was 48.5).

"The gynae could have led with that," I thought.

The next day I phoned my daughter's surgeon in Cape Town. He was a brilliant doctor and like my friend Elaine an extraordinary compassionate person.

He agreed that a CT scan was necessary.

The radiologist kindly tried to distract me with a political discussion. It worked for a few minutes, but then she left the room and the terror returned as I held my breath while my body was pushed through the machine. As I left, I peeked into the control room where two women were looking at the images of my pelvis. "Please give me good news," I pleaded – hoping that my request could change the outcome.

The surgeon called 30 minutes later. There was some good and some bad news. There were no signs of any spreading, but there was a growth, and it was huge – bigger than initially thought.

"It has to be removed, or it will start putting pressure on other organs. Frankly, I'm surprised that you haven't had more discomfort," he said gently.

After the call, I wondered if I had missed anything. I had for the previous two months felt some bladder discomfort. My GP ruled out a urinary tract infection and suggested that it might be linked to menopause – the go-to for everything at my age it, seems. She prescribed an oestrogen cream which had given me some relief, but from time to time there had still been a dull pain low down on my right side. Was that it?

My daughter's surgeon referred me to another doctor who specialised in ovarian issues. Sitting in the waiting room, I felt like an imposter. He was part of a bigger fertility practice, and the place was filled with young couples full of hope. I was not only about three decades older, but I was on my own, as instructed by the receptionist on account of COVID.

Another internal ultrasound was needed. I tried to ignore the discomfort by focussing on the bit of the specialist's face visible above his face mask. I could see his frown deepen as he moved the probe deeper and in different directions. It hurt. He apologised. He did an internal exam with his fingers. It hurt. He apologised. He went back to the ultrasound again. By now my legs were shaking violently. I felt cold and sore, and the terror was growing.

"I'm not sure, but I think there is a second tumour, and I see some free-flowing fluid. We don't like to see that," he said as he pointed to the dark images on the ultrasound.

The dam wall started to collapse.

"How did they not see it on the CT scan?" I asked.

"They sometimes miss things, depending on how you were lying. In any case, I would do you a disservice if I operate on you. You need to go and see a gynaecological oncologist – the best one in town".

Sitting across from him, I felt nauseous with panic. Things had now moved from "I might have cancer" to "I most probably have cancer."

Walking to my car, I felt my legs buckle.

"I really want to live to see my grandchildren," was all I could think as I sobbed while driving home.

The next day, Prof Hennie Botha, head of gynaecological oncology at Stellenbosch University, saw me. By now it was clear that surgery was going to be required, the only question was by whom and what would be removed.

I also knew that I needed to trust and like the person who was going to cut into me. "If I don't like this guy, I reserve the right to look for someone else," I said to a friend before the appointment.

Luckily, I immediately liked the Professor. We had been at Stellenbosch University at the same time. We shared similar historical reference points, and I knew his cousins. Even though I have no deep attachment to Afrikaans, it was strangely comforting that he spoke in my mother tongue.

"I'm usually very mind over matter, but I feel like my dog when there is a thunderstorm," I opened up to him. "I'm frantically trying to find a place to hide to make this go away, but everywhere I go, it is still there."

After another ultrasound – this time thankfully an external one – he took my hand and pressed it next to my bellybutton. There it was – the thing that had quietly grown in me during the last 12 months. (There had been no sign of any abnormality during my previous gynaecological visit).

After I got dressed, he showed me the images of the CT scan. My jaw dropped. "All of that?" I whispered, looking at the huge white circle crowding out other organs.

Prof Botha gently explained my options, but also did not mince his words. The chance of the growth being cancerous was at least 70%.

"You don't have to use me, but it has to come out and soon," he said.

"Are you good?" I asked while monitoring his reaction closely. He paused, thought for a few seconds and then calmly looked me in the eyes.

"Yes, I am good."

Two days later he held my hand as the general anaesthetic took effect and 90 minutes later, he again squeezed my hand as he assured me that all had gone well. He had taken out the growth – all 9 cm in diameter and 190 grams of it. I was now also without a cervix, ovaries, uterus and omentum (the lining that protects our digestive system where cancer cells like to "hide".)

The final verdict on whether it was cancer would take a few days...

Still Hurts Like Hell!

"Wow! The anaesthetist was kind to you," said one of the medical personnel looking at my chart.

"Why?" I asked.

"Well, I see he prescribed three days of intravenous paracetamol. We don't usually prescribe the good stuff for that long after a hysterectomy."

"Why? Is it dangerous?" I asked.

"No," he replied.

After he left, I felt a mixture of confused shame.

"Am I weak?" I wondered. "Should I have been off the drip already, even though it still hurts like hell?"

Three days earlier I had fought my way back from the darkness of anaesthesia. It felt like my belly was on fire. The pain was excruciating. All I could whisper was "pain, pain" when asked how I was doing for the first hour after the operation.

My body was also shaking violently with what I would later discover was a desperate attempt to try and regulate my temperature after two hours under anaesthesia.

For the first night, I was given a morphine pump to self-administer. However, I hated the feeling of morphine and was started on intravenous paracetamol the next day. Although not as strong as morphine, it helped enormously while my pain receptors were still in overdrive.

Early on day two I was also encouraged to get out of bed. Relying on my years of Pilates training, I took a deep breath, tried to engage my core and slowly stood up.

"It feels like someone had torn open my stomach and removed my insides," I grimaced at the nurse. "That's exactly what they did," she responded, not spotting my sarcasm.

Back in bed, sweating and out of breath from another few minutes of painful exertion, I thought again about the doctor's comment.

"How could three days of IV paracetamol be regarded as kind?" I wondered. "I have a scar that runs from just below my belly button to my pubic bone. They had cut through multiple layers of skin, muscle, tendons and blood vessels to remove numerous organs. Surely a few days of strong painkillers was acceptable? It was, after all, paracetamol and not some form of an addictive opiate?"

Still, I couldn't shake the thought that I was not a model patient or that I wasn't tough enough.

After three nights in hospital, I was discharged. I was given a prescription for paracetamol and ibuprofen for pain management.

"How long should I use this?" I asked one of the surgeons.

"About three days," he answered. "Or longer if you can't manage."

Again, the message seemed really ambiguous.

I have often been told that I have a high pain threshold. I very rarely take painkillers. A few years ago, I broke my little finger in three places, and despite the hand specialist describing it as "a very serious break," I only took painkillers twice.

Yet, the pain of the hysterectomy was worse than anything (including C-sections and a breast operation) I had experienced before. To get into bed was painful. To get out of bed was worse. To turn around in bed required gripping the bed sheets for support. To bend down was impossible.

It also lasted for weeks (some pain stayed for months) and not days as the instructions on the prescription seemed to suggest. The pain was unpleasant to deal with, but it was aggravated by the feelings of doubt and shame.

Still feeling extremely sore and unwell on day ten, I turned to Google. I came across an open letter a woman called Kate Hale wrote after her laparoscopic hysterectomy.[1]
On day ten, I am lying here in bed fighting the tears because I know I have to take a pain pill to just be able to relax," she wrote. "I didn't imagine this simple outpatient

---

[1] https://www.youbrewmytea.com/10-days-after-hysterectomy-with-one-regret/

surgery could leave me so completely drained. Let alone hurting so deeply for so long."

Below Kate's moving piece a string of comments from women told of their pain and confusion post-surgery:

"I am on day six and keep questioning why I am not feeling better."

"Weirdest and most painful surgery I have ever had. I told everyone I would be up and about after 3 weeks ...lying in bed now still having pain...like sore body nauseous...pain in my abdomen area... with my laptop besides me having meetings online to attend important stuff yet my body hurts."

"I had my laparoscopic total hysterectomy only two days ago and woke up early this morning just feeling terrible. I've not been taking Rx pain meds except before bed (to help me sleep, really) but have also been taking high strength OTC pain meds. Then just now, upon waking early am, I wanted to cry, I'm so sore, achy."

"I needed to hear this. I have tears in my eyes, although it hurts to even cry because your stomach jumps up and down, but I needed to hear this. All I have done is cry, take short naps, drink ice water, fight with my husband because he's not emotionally here for me and has attempted to physically not be here for me, be nauseous, dizzy at times, mouth dry from Percocet, and yes attempt to do my woman/motherly duties since no one can do it right except me! This procedure is nothing like I have expected.

Yes, I too believed that after 3-4 days I would've felt better and planned on going back to work in two weeks."

What struck me was not only how much pain the women endured, but that, like me, they thought that they were supposed to feel less or even no pain. All of them conveyed a sense of shame for not being up and fulfilling their normal duties, even though it was just days after major surgery.

To be fair to the surgeon, he did warn beforehand that during week one I would be mostly in bed. During week two, he said, I would be wanting to be more on the couch and by week three I would be ready to make myself a sandwich.

I can now say for certain that from my and many other women's experience of (especially) abdominal hysterectomies, it was a drastic overestimation of the speed of recovery.

It took about three months to be relatively pain free. More than a year later, l would still feel the occasional pull around the scar. It took at least eight months to feel physically more like myself again.

When I mentioned my level of discomfort to a friend who is a general surgeon a few weeks after the operation, he nodded and said: "That is understandable. A radical, abdominal hysterectomy is one of the biggest operations we do."

His words gave me some comfort, but I could not help wondering why that message was not conveyed more clearly to women, both in terms of recovery time and pain relief. Between tortuous visits to the bathroom, I started to look for answers.

I stumbled across a book called *Doing Harm: The truth about how bad medicine and lazy science leave women dismissed, misdiagnosed and sick*, by Maya Dusenbery.[2] This phenomenal book reveals how the vast majority of medical research is done on male bodies and thus often inappropriate when it comes to treating women with similar conditions. Dusenbery calls the fact that medical science knows less of "every aspect of the female biology compared to male biology"[3] the knowledge gap. However, what really interested me was what she called the trust gap.

Dusenbery points to research that has proven that doctors don't take women's complaints as seriously as those of men. For example, studies revealed that women wait, on average, 65 minutes compared to men's 45 minutes to get treatment for abdominal pain in the emergency room in America. They were also less likely to be given strong painkillers such as opiates despite having the same pain scores as male patients.[4] Other research proved that

---

[2] Harper Collins, 2018.

[3] Location 230

[4] Chen EH, Shofer FS, Dean AJ, et al. Gender disparity in analgesic treatment of emergency department patients with acute abdominal pain. Acad Emerg Med. 2008;15(5):414-418

women were seven times more likely to be sent home in the middle of a heart attack than men.[5]

Deborah Copaken, in her book *Ladyparts,* says that when a woman claims that her pain is seven out of ten, her doctor will assume it is five, while men's self-reported pain is taken as face value. [6]

This is borne out by research. A recent study found that medical doctors believed that female patients had less pain and were more likely to exaggerate pain. This resulted in men being far more likely to be recommended pain relief, while women were recommended psychological treatment.[7]

In addition − or perhaps because of this gender bias − women tend to underplay their physical complaints in fear of being seen as emotional or hysterical. Copaken describes why she minimised her serious medical condition for years: "Society teaches us (women) to minimise our woes and to internalise its sceptical view of our pain so as not to be labelled cry-babies or 'hysterical': a meaningless diagnosis of unspecified female malaise, which in the nineteenth or twentieth centuries, could sometimes mean you'd walk out of the doctor's office minus a clitoris."[8]

Wanting to sound stoic or brave, I know that I have also done that for years.

___

[5] Dusenbery, Loc 103
[6] Deborah Copaken, Ladyparts, Random House, 2021, p.20
[7] Schäfer G, et al. Health care providers' judgments in chronic pain: The influence of gender and trustworthiness. Pain. 2016;157(8):1618-1625.
[8] Copaken, p.20

It was now also clear to me that women faced a double whammy when it came to pain management. When asked about her level of pain, a woman will often describe it as a six or a five even though it feels like a seven. Her physician would then either consciously or sub-consciously take that as an exaggeration and classify the pain as a four or three and base pain relief on this wholly inadequate rating.

The "kindness" of three days paracetamol started to make sense.

Many women would later tell me similar stories.

One friend related how she had a long, difficult labour without any pain relief. After eight hours she eventually had a suction assisted birth, which necessitated an episiotomy (a surgical cut between the vagina and anus or perineum) with multiple layers of stitches.

Unsurprisingly, she felt very sore afterwards and asked for some pain relief. Intravenous paracetamol was prescribed. The next morning, only hours after the birth and episiotomy, the doctor came to see her. She watched as he looked at her chart, took out his red pen and drew a line through the instruction for IV paracetamol. "That's enough of that now. It's total overkill for an episiotomy," he said firmly.

My friend, who by the way is a medical doctor with a background in obstetrics, said she thought afterwards of many things she should have said to him such as: "Have you ever had your perineum cut and stitched up again?" or "Would you really have said that to a man with a similar injury?" Instead, believing that she was not tough enough, she felt intense shame and confusion – as I did.

I had not anticipated, nor was I warned about how exhausting and lengthy the physical recovery process would be. I was not prepared for the bloating (it lasted months), the painful bladder functions (also months), the constipation (luckily only for a few days), the fact that some internal stitches might never dissolve (the painful pokes lasted a year) and that I would be out of breath and energy for months.

It was intensely messy, confusing and scary.

It was also lonely. After five weeks I was signed off by the surgeon. From a medical or surgical point of view it was all over. Except it wasn't.

It had only really started.

Grief

I stared at the photo.

There on a green theatre cloth lay my ovaries, uterus and cervix. Pink and beautiful just like they would have been inside me. Except, on the right ovary was the growth. A huge, angry, brain-like thing – complete with veins and big knobs.

The surgeon had asked permission to take photos during the operation and shortly after asked if I wanted to see it.

Only late on day three did I feel brave enough to look at it. I was alone in the four-bed ward, and it was uncharacteristically quiet. Struggling to sleep, I took out my phone and scrolled to the photo.

Earlier that day, Prof Botha had called. "I have good news," he said. "The growth was rare, but totally benign!"

I waited for relief to come.

It didn't.

I felt like I had to thank him.

I couldn't.

"But we removed all those organs," I said, my voice shaking. "Did we make a mistake?"

He explained that we had no choice, that the fibroma (it now had a name) was rare (only 3-4% of all ovarian tumours are fibromas, which are by definition benign) and that the chance that it would have been a cancerous tumour instead had been extremely high.

"If we had not removed all the organs, and the pathologist had found just one rogue cell under the microscope, we would have had to go back into theatre today, open you up again and remove it all. That would not have been good. Now rest and be happy," he said, before saying goodbye.

My rational brain berated my heart. I should be thankful that there would be no chemotherapy, no radiation – that I would live to see my grandchildren.

This was a fantastic outcome and after all, I had no need for those organs anymore.

But my heart felt otherwise

Later that evening, in the orange circle of the bed light, I stared at the photo.

Since I was 13 years old these organs were a constant reminder of what made me a woman.

Every 28 days, I would feel the rise in sexual tension as an egg travelled from my ovaries through the fallopian tubes. This would be followed by an irritation-filled build-up to the arrival of my period. A few days later my uterus would shed the lining which she diligently prepared in anticipation of a pregnancy. I once calculated that I had menstruated about 356 times in my life – 2492 days, seven years in total.

I zoomed into the photo to look more closely at my uterus. I tried to imagine how the perfectly round little ball had stretched to provide a safe space for my babies to grow. First for my daughter 31 years before, and then my son two years later. I tried to see the scars of the C-sections, but clearly this amazing organ had repaired herself fully in anticipation of more arrivals.

I studied my cervix. This mouth-like structure, which provided the entry way for my babies to the world and yet protected my internal organs from onslaughts from a germ-filled external environment. I was filled with tender awe. She looked beautiful and yet so strong.

Then the implications of what happened hit me...

My beautiful uterus, ovaries and cervix were no longer part of me. They were in a bottle full of preservatives, somewhere in a lab – ready to be dissected, after which they would be thrown into a bag of medical waste and incinerated. They were on their final journey – a journey my body would follow sometime in the future.

The grief suddenly overwhelmed me, and deep sobs shook my body. I wanted to say thank you, to hold them, to put them back ... but it was too late.

Over the next few weeks, I was absorbed with physical healing. It was exhausting and all consuming, yet I knew that the grief was hovering somewhere in the background.

At night it would rise from my subconscious into my dreams – unsurprisingly in the form of Gerry.

Gerry Ryan was the love of my life. He was an extraordinary man – larger than life, funny, generous and kind. And for a short while he was mine. We first met when he interviewed me shortly after I had arrived in Dublin to take up my position as South African Ambassador.

For me it was just another interview, but he later admitted that he had decided then that if I was ever free in the future, he would pursue me.

A few years later I was hosting a radio programme at the national broadcaster where he had for over 20 years presented a daily three-hour show. He saw that my hair colour had changed and suspected that it was indicative of bigger changes in my life.

He was right. My marriage of almost 20 years had reached a painful end.

He made contact. At first, I resisted. After being married for most of my adult life to a man with a well-known surname, I was not keen to go down that road again. Yet, if Gerry set his eye on something, he didn't give up easily.

After much persuasion, I finally agreed to meet him at his penthouse for a drink. By the end of the night, I had fallen hopelessly in love with him and for the next two years we would be deliriously happy...

Then on 30 April 2010, I found his lifeless body on our

bedroom floor and at that moment my long, excruciatingly painful journey of grief started.

It came as no surprise that my post-operative dreams were filled with Gerry. Soon after I got home, I dreamt – as I often did in the year after his death – that he was alive, that he had never died. In the dream I was somewhere in Ireland and suddenly saw him amongst a crowd of people. He spotted me and – as he had done in real life – gave me a beaming smile whilst opening his arms wide. Overjoyed, I ran to him, and he folded me into his big, black coat, the one we had bought in New York together. When I woke up from the dream, I could smell his scent, feel the sensation of his coat against my face. My body ached for him. I needed him to help me through this – to make everything right again.

I wept as I tried to roll myself into a foetus position, but pulling up my legs resulted in excruciating pain, so I just sobbed.

Grief is funny thing. It is something only those who have walked a similar road can fully understand. It also never leaves you completely.

As a woman in Ireland told me decades after her husband's death: "Grief is like a handbag that you pick up the day your loved one dies and you can never put it down again. The best you can hope for is that with time the handbag becomes lighter and that you might eventually – for a little while – forget that you are carrying it. "

Over the years, my handbag of grief had indeed become

lighter – even though it was still rare for a day to pass without me thinking of Gerry.

Would the lessons I learnt help me now?

A few weeks earlier I had read an article in the New Yorker by the Nigerian author, Chimamanda Ngozi Adichie. In "Notes on Grief" she wrote movingly about her experience after her father died.

"Is this what shock means, that the air turns to glue?" she asks, and I know exactly what she means.

Air turning into glue… when even breathing becomes painful.

It took about eight weeks before my body started to feel a bit better and it was then that the question from George, my vet, triggered the full emotional cascade of grief again.

Over the next few months, I struggled through glue-like air as I walked the familiar path of grief and recovery once more and remembered the important road marks from the past.

The first step was to give into the sadness. It was there and no matter how hard I tried to rationalise it away with I-did-not-need-those-organs-anymore thoughts, it was not going to go away. In fact, it would get stronger.

I also had to accept that it was ok to be sad. I had lost organs – and not just any organs – those that were so key to my identity as a woman.

I had to remind myself that recovery is different for everyone and that I had to choose carefully who I looked to for support. When my mum mentioned that my dad went back to work the day after she came home after her hysterectomy and she "just had to get on with things", it sent me into a terrible shame cycle. My Pilates instructor's remark that some of his other clients were able to do Pilates two weeks post-operative had me in tears.

In contrast, a women's circle once a month was one of the most important places of healing. The group of deeply compassionate women understood intuitively that this was a big deal. They listened and cried with me. In the strange cyberworld of COVID, they "held" my grief over thousands of kilometres from all corners of the world.

They helped me to remember that the journey of grief has its own timetable and that it would take as long as it took. A psychologist once told me that mourning was the only process that they could not speed up through therapeutic interventions. "All we can do is be there and hold people's hands along the way".

I had to also accept that the eight-weeks sick leave certificate only applied to the physical recovery (and not really even that). In fact, it was the imminent end to the sick leave that triggered the full-blown grief.

Although I resisted it at first, I knew I needed to find help... from the right people. Soon after the operation, I spoke for hours to an amazing healing therapist. Wendy had had a double mastectomy and full hysterectomy after being diagnosed with aggressive breast cancer at a young age.

Although she was careful in sharing her story, it helped me tremendously to know that she understood in every possible sense what I was going through.

I also spoke to my friend Abraham, who is an amazing therapist, and later I did work with a deeply empathetic osteopath.

What surprised me most was that the operation triggered a cascade of old traumas and fears. Long after the wounds from the operation healed, my body and mind demanded that I look carefully at the dark corners of my psyche and life.

It would be a deeply uncomfortable but rewarding journey to freedom.

Rage

The feeling unsettled me. It was so intense that I wondered if I should stop the car.

Only a few days earlier I was cleared for driving and I was delighted to be free to move around on my own again. Although I'm not particularly fond of driving, I have often made deep emotional and intellectual breakthroughs in the cocoonlike space of a car or airplane.

Years ago, for example, I was struggling to figure out what to do next in my life. I was no longer happy as a member of parliament and my marriage was in serious trouble. I was exhausted beyond belief and struggling with my health.

One day on a long drive to visit a part of my constituency, I was praying to God, the universe ... anybody...to help me.

It was a hot, clear summer day and the road stretched out for miles in front of me. Just after I sent my silent prayer up, a huge misty cloud suddenly appeared on the road in front of me. It was bizarre. "If ever I would get a vision, this would be it," I thought.

I drove into the cloud and for a few seconds I was enfolded by a light grey mist. There was no vision. I exited, feeling slightly disappointed. Then suddenly a thought – as clear as the bright sunlight outside came into my mind: "You should go to Ireland!"

"What?" I said aloud to myself.

"You should become ambassador," another clear thought.

Although I had no idea where these thoughts came from, I immediately felt enormous peace and clarity.

In the days that followed, it turned out that there was a vacancy in the Embassy in Dublin, the head of the foreign service said he would be delighted to have me as long as the President agreed, and lo and behold, the president agreed not only to see me, but also to my request.

A few months later my family and I were on our way to Ireland, where I would spend the next twelve – life altering – years of my life.

So, I had learned to pay attention to sudden big feelings when I'm driving.

I felt my hands sweating and my heart racing.

What was happening?

I dropped into the feeling and then it dawned on me. It was rage. Not irritation or indignation – or even anger. It was a boiling, red-hot RAGE.

I had just spent an hour with a deeply empathetic functional doctor who had for the previous two years helped me to get through menopause. Erika had moved into functional medicine after a very traumatic birth of her first child.

Her, "I'm so sorry for what had happened to you" greeting had immediately opened the flood gates and for an hour I relayed the shock, pain, powerlessness and fear of the previous weeks.

After an hour of crying, I was spent, but a lot calmer as I got into the car. There was a momentary emptiness inside of me and it felt good. Of course, unless you are the Dalai Lama or Thich Nhaht Hanh, emotional emptiness does not last long.

So, ten minutes later, rage filled the space created by the momentary calmness.

I wasn't completely surprised. There had been little warning signs of this imminent eruption. On the day I left hospital, I had questioned the surgeon about the effect of the drop of hormone levels after the removal of my ovaries. He casually (or so it seemed to me) remarked about a possible loss of libido.

I immediately saw red.

"You would never say that so casually to a man," I said angrily. "If this was a male issue, the medical world would find a solution.... oh wait, but you have. A little blue pill!"

To be fair, the surgeon did offer some solutions, but this was only the preamble to what was to become a personal and political fury.

A few days earlier, the same surgeon had remarked on the difficulties in diagnosing ovarian cancer. At that stage, I already knew that the CA-125 blood test for tumour markers was very unreliable for an initial diagnosis. (It is more useful in the detection of a return of ovarian cancer following treatment).

The other diagnostic tools available are ultrasounds, CT and MRI scans. Ultrasounds are unclear and usually only signal a growth or thickness, while CT and MRI scans will reveal whether it is a fluid filled mass (more indicative of a cyst – and thus less problematic) or a hard mass (and thus more concerning).

However, all three specialists I had consulted had explained that the only way to definitively know whether a hard mass is malignant is surgery. If there is any suspicion that it might be cancerous, they will usually opt for abdominal or open surgery (as opposed to laparoscopic or vaginal procedure) in order to prevent any potential cells "chipping off" during the operation and "seeding" amongst your remaining organs.

In most cases they also have to send the growth away for a thorough laboratory analysis – so can't just make a call on the nature of the tumour in theatre.

As explained by the surgeon on the day I got my results, if there is any suspicion of a possible malignancy, as a matter of caution they tend to favour a hysterectomy in order to avoid another surgery shortly after.

So, even though the surgeon presented me with various options prior to the surgery, the only real choice was between a radical hysterectomy or possible death. Which of course is not really a choice.

Six weeks later in the car, I suddenly had a vivid image of women all over the world with deep red scars on their abdomens, struggling to heal emotionally and physically from hysterectomies.

How archaic and brutal!!

How was it possible that in this age when we can transplant hearts, do the most sophisticated brain operations and even perform surgical procedures on babies before birth, we have no way of figuring out if a woman has ovarian cancer except to cut her open and rip out all her reproductive organs?

In fact, a doctor would later tell me that hysterectomies were the only routine (as opposed to trauma related) open abdominal surgeries still done today.

When I got home, I grabbed my laptop.

First, I had to get the definitions right. Although the word hysterectomy is often used in a general sense to describe removal of women's reproductive organs, it strictly means the removal of the uterus (It comes from the Greek word "Hustera", which means womb.) The removal of ovaries is referred to as an oophorectomy as opposed to a radical trachelectomy or cervicectomy which is the removal of the cervix. A radical hysterectomy generally means the removal of the ovaries, uterus and cervix. This is what I had.

As with many other surgeries, the history of hysterectomies does not make for pleasant reading.

Vaginal hysterectomies were apparently even performed in ancient times, and as one would expect, they were brutal. Good old Soranus of Ephesus, who lived in 120 BC, basically pulled out the uterus through the vagina. This practice continued through the Middle Ages. Unsurprisingly women rarely (my guess is never) survived the procedure. Until the discovery of antibiotics, anaesthesia and blood transfusions, the mortality rate remained around 70%.

According to some articles I read, the first successful (meaning the woman didn't die) abdominal hysterectomy was performed in 1929 by a Dr Richardson. Believe it or not, there were very few advances in the following fifty years until the development of laparoscopic surgery.[9]

As it goes with Google, I was heading down a rabbit hole. I found article after article talking about how many unnecessary hysterectomies were performed around the world. In the USA, for example, it is the second most common surgery for women. About 600 000 are performed every year, only 10% of them for cancer diagnoses.[10] Another study revealed that 70% of hysterectomies did not meet an expert physician panel's

---

[9]

https://www.sciencedirect.com/science/article/abs/pii/S0950355297800478

[10] https://lowninstitute.org/guest-post-the-madness-of-unnecessary-hysterectomy-has-to-stop/

criteria for hysterectomy and 76% did not meet criteria established by the American College of Obstetricians and Gynaecologists (ACOG).[11] There were similar studies in the UK.

As shocking as that was, I had to remind myself that I was one of the 10% that required a cancer diagnosis, and that therefore, my procedure was not done lightly. Still, if there had been better tools available to diagnose ovarian cancer, they could have removed only the one ovary – a much simpler and less invasive procedure with fewer long-term consequences. (I had to stop reading about the long-term effects, since I was rapidly running the risk of a severe depression).

Unsurprisingly the answer lay in the discrepancy in research funding. In the United Kingdom, only 2.5% of publicly funded research is dedicated to female reproductive health, despite the fact that one out of three women will suffer reproductive health problems.

According to the American Cancer Association. Ovarian cancer ranks fifth in cancer deaths among women, accounting for more deaths than any other cancer of the female reproductive system.

Yet, between 2013 and 2018, the National Cancer Institute allocated $611 million for ovarian cancer research, compared to almost $1.5 billion (2 ½ times as much) for prostate cancer research. The numbers for cervical and

---

[11] https://www.webmd.com/women/news/20000131/more-hysterectomies-more-inappropriate-reasons

uterine cancer were even less than ovarian cancer. Numbers were similar in Canada and the UK.

Elisabeth Baugh, CEO of Ovarian Cancer Canada[12], pointed out that ovarian cancer is the most fatal gynaecological cancer in Canada. Yet, almost three times more money is spent on research into prostate cancer than ovarian cancer there – even though the five-year survival rate for prostate cancer is between 90% and 100%). She also pointed out that ovarian cancer survival rates hadn't improved in 50 years because of a significant underfunding of research in this area.

If that wasn't enough, it also turns out that there is five times more funded research into erectile dysfunction (which affects 19% of men) than into premenstrual syndrome, which affects 90% of women.

After about an hour, I closed my laptop and lay down in a bundle of exhausted fury.

Over the next few weeks, the anger would grow. Every time I looked at the angry red and painful scar on my stomach, I would feel the rage growing inside me.

It went far beyond just the inequality of medical research. It was as if the scar became a symbol of the deeper wound to women around the world.

---

[12] https://www.globenewswire.com/news-release/2018/02/28/1401168/0/en/Budget-2018-Ovarian-cancer-research-funding-still-a-concern-for-women.html

It was as if the removal of my female organs lifted a veil and everywhere I looked I saw with renewed clarity the terrible injustice done to women.

Unsurprising the physical became political – again.

The physical is political

I live in a country with some of the worst gender-based violence anywhere on earth. When confronted on a daily basis with horrendous stories, it is natural to start blocking it out in order not to get too petrified to go out your front door (or in many cases go in through the front door). Every so often there are stories that you can't block out – they are just so shocking that they demand your full attention.

Early one morning, about a month after my operation, the press started to report that body parts were found in a suitcase on a pavement in a city called East London. As the day went on it became clear that the body parts were female. A few hours later, following a trail of blood, the police arrested a man. He readily admitted to killing and dismembering his girlfriend, because, he claimed, she was having an affair. The victim was Nosicelo Mtebeni, a 23-year-old final year law student. She was the first one in her family to go to university and had big dreams.

I know that most people would assume that the killer had serious mental health issues. The thing is that he didn't. He claimed that he just got angry – pushed and hit her (which he clearly thought he was justified in doing) and she died.

This is not an exceptional case. Thousands of women in my country get killed by their partners or family members every year.

During the same time, there was a case in court of a man

who paid some men to kill his seven-months pregnant girlfriend. She was found hanging from a tree.

A few days after Nosicelo's death made headlines, someone sent me figures released by the Department of Health in one of our nine provinces. In that province alone, there were 23000 teenage pregnancies in 12 months. Some were as young as 10 years of age.

I felt sick to my stomach. These girls were still babies themselves. Not only were they raped and abused by older men, they were also facing very dangerous pregnancies that could result in death or serious physical harm. They would in all likelihood drop out of school and so the cycle of poverty would continue.

As in most countries around the world, having sex with anyone under the age of sixteen is illegal in South Africa and deemed to be sexual assault or rape. Still, the relevant cabinet minister passed the buck by saying that law enforcement was not her department's responsibility, so she could not say whether anyone was prosecuted.

I was livid.

Then Texas hit the headlines. The Texas state legislature in the USA, comprised of 73% (mostly white older) men, passed a law that would prohibit abortions in that state as soon as what resembles a heartbeat could be detected on a sonogram. This could be as early as six weeks after conception, before most women would even suspect that they might be pregnant. It even applies in the case of a pregnancy following incest or rape.

To make matters worse, the law opened the door for almost any private citizen to sue abortion providers and even incentivises such litigation by rewarding the litigants with $10,000 and legal costs in the case of a successful prosecution.

This was only the preamble to much worse to come. Months later the US Supreme Court would overturn the decades old Roe v Wade decision, which gave the green light to many states to bring in draconian legislation regarding women's reproductive health.

How was it possible that after all these years of fighting, we were seeing such terrible reversals in progress for women?

Surely it was clear to everyone what the inevitable outcome would be? Women who could afford it would travel to another state where abortions were legal (as rapidly happened with Texan women traveling to Oklahoma). Those without the resources would have no choice but to resort to back street abortions and in doing so risk their lives and of course prosecution.

Yet, these men, none of whom had ever given birth (and I doubt many of them had ever changed a diaper), triumphantly declared that they were "saving thousands of God-given lives."

My wonderful Jamaican friend, Nadine, always says: "If you really want to hit at the core of a society, you get in between a women's legs."

So true!

I knew that all of this would have annoyed me before my operation, but now I felt a familiar angry determination stirring inside me – something I had buried for a few decades.

I am not new to gender battles. As a theology student, I was for three years the only woman in my class of over 50 men. Within days after arriving on campus, I raised the unfairness of a curfew for female students who lived in residence, with the head of the university. "It is for your own protection," he said patronizingly. "You know what men are like."

"Then, why don't you lock up the men?" I asked angrily.

I eventually did a Master's degree on the topic of feminist theology – despite resistance from the head of faculty. "No one takes feminism seriously as an academic field," he insisted when I presented him with the topic of my thesis.

A few years later I was the youngest woman to be elected to the first democratic parliament of South Africa. For the first time ever there were now more than 100 female MPs. Even though we were almost one third of all the members, it did not translate into a supportive or even equitable workspace.

Childcare was a battle only won after we brought all our children to parliament one day. The chaos it caused focussed the attention of the mostly male civil servants. Maternity leave took years to organise. Female toilets were scarce and after weeks of asking for more toilets to be designated to women nothing had happened.

So, we took matters into our own hands, replaced the door signs and put plants into the urinals.

On a more personal level I was often asked by senior male colleagues to type things for them or book plane tickets. I was also once dropped from a panel that I had worked very hard to get onto, after I declined a minister's request to go home with him one night. "My wife is away and I'm lonely," he said.

Seven years later, I was the youngest ambassador to be appointed. Diplomacy remains an (elderly) male dominated world. So throughout my four years as Ambassador, I would be looked up and down at the endless cocktail parties by male colleagues and told: "You look hopelessly too young to be an ambassador and you're a woman!"

I usually responded with: "Yes, they tried the old men, but it hasn't worked out so well. So now they are giving us younger women a chance."

I wasn't really made for diplomacy.

At one conference in rural Ireland, all the speakers (who with the exception of myself were male) were introduced at the beginning of the conference. When it came to me, the presenter said: "Melanie Verwoerd is South Africa's ambassador." He paused and looked over at me.

"Stand up love," he said.

No one else had been asked to stand, but not wanting to make a fuss I stood up and gave a little wave to the audience.

Before I could sit down, the presenter said: "Now give us a twirl, love. Go on, let them have a good look at you."

I was gobsmacked. "Surely I had misunderstood," I thought. However, seeing him making a little circle sign with his hand made me realise I had not.

"No!" I said angrily and sat down. An uncomfortable silence fell in the hall.

Later the room fell silent when I made reference to sexist nature of it in my speech. Needless to say, I was never invited back.

So, for years, I studied and lived feminism. I was an activist and I fought men and their patriarchal attitudes. As the years went by, my beliefs did not change, nor the anger I felt when I was faced with the many injustices women had (and have) to deal with. Yet, I became less of an activist. I had babies to raise, money to make and a marriage to keep together.

Yet, now, it felt like something was shifting. It was as if this physical crisis had lifted a veil. I wasn't sure where it would take me, but I knew I had no choice but to open the veil and bravely walk through.

I knew it would be a journey of not only physical and emotional healing after the hysterectomy, but also of the deeper wounds I – and many women – carry.

I knew it was not going to be easy – especially since it was within the context of the world's own collective crisis.

We are all grieving

About five months after the operation, I was chatting to a friend on the phone, when I absentmindedly rubbed my shin. I froze. There was a lump. I rubbed again – trying to feel if it was loose or attached. I couldn't get it to move.

I felt intense panic rise. Not again!!

I tried hard to talk myself down and after the phone conversation ended, I phoned the GP and made an appointment.

The GP prodded around and suggested an ultra-sound to figure out what it was. I could only get a booking three days later and despite my best intentions to stay calm, it was difficult not to relive the events of a few months earlier.

"Was this now what my life was going to be like – one health scare after the other?" I wondered.

Sitting in the radiologist's waiting room a few days later, I overheard the woman next to me talking to the receptionist about a recent CT scan.

"It sounds like you have been through the wars already," I gently said to her. She was clearly delighted to talk. It turns out she was a medical doctor who had earlier in the year contracted COVID from one of her patients. She eventually ended up in ICU and was now suffering from long-term COVID with many debilitating symptoms.

When I was called for my test, I wished her well. I was met by two lovely women who welcomed me cheerfully. "Look, I have a bit of PTSD," I said and then explained what had happened earlier in the year.

The two women were exceptionally empathetic and while one moved the ultra-sound probe over my leg, the older of two revealed that she also had a hysterectomy a few months earlier.

With the story of the doctor in the waiting room still very much in my mind, I asked the two radiologists how they had coped through COVID.

"It was hard, so hard" said the one.

"With the fear of infection?" I asked.

"Not so much that, it was when we had to go up to scan the seriously sick COVID patients in ICU. You could see the fear in their eyes, but there was no one there for them. No one touching them, no one just saying: 'it's ok, it's ok'."

Her eyes welled up for a moment.

"You know I said to myself: 'what the hell!' I knew I wasn't supposed to touch them, but I couldn't bear it anymore. So, I would take their hands and rub their arms and tell them to be strong. It broke my heart."

She wiped away a few tears. Then she turned to me.

"Darling, I can feel the lump, but I can't see anything on the screen. I'm sure it's just a fatty deposit."

She smiled. "You know this is the problem after a hysterectomy. You can't let yourself go. The fat goes everywhere. See what has happened to you? Fat is now even sitting below your knees."

We all burst out laughing.

Driving back home, I felt a huge sense of relief. I also felt grateful for these two empathetic, humorous women, who understood my anxiety.

Still, the conversations with both the doctor in the waiting room and the radiologists again emphasized the terrible time we were living in with COVID.

On 14 March 2020 our own journey with COVID started with a phone call.

"Mum, I think I'm really ill."

My usually unflappable daughter's voice was shaking on the other side of the phone and even though there were only five confirmed cases at that stage in South Africa, I knew something big was wrong.

A week of celebrations with over 50 of her friends from all over the world had culminated in a joyous wedding the day before and the newlyweds had set off on a short honeymoon.

Three days later the results were in. She had tested positive for COVID-19. By that stage my whole family and a number of wedding guests were ill. My son and I had relatively mild symptoms, but my daughter was not so lucky. Thankfully her new husband is a paramedic and could keep a close eye on her vitals as her fever was raging and the virus moved to her chest. Not the best of starts for a marriage.

Fourteen days later we were finally cleared to leave quarantine. That night the President announced that South Africa would go into level 5 lockdown. Only essential services were open, we had a curfew from 8 pm till 6 am and no one was allowed to be outside their homes, unless it was to visit grocery shops, doctors or other essential services.

A few hours before lockdown was due to kick in, I quickly drove to my sister's house to deliver little trees that her kids wanted to plant. In return she was to lend me some ridiculously complicated puzzles. My sister had her elderly father in-law staying with her and (rightly so) didn't want to take any chances. So she left the puzzles outside the gate and we shouted a brief hallo from two meters away in the dark, while my darling little nephews hovered at the back.

As I drove away, I had a little meltdown. It had been fifteen days of isolation and the idea of another three weeks (it ended up being three months and eventually another 18 months of some form of lockdown) felt just too much as I struggled with the image of my sister and nephews behind a gate. The streets were eerily quiet, and I became overwhelmed with fear of what could happen in the next few weeks in the country I love so much. I wept as I prayed that not too many people would die.

At home, I told myself to get a grip, since I had so much to be thankful for. My family had survived the virus, my house is comfortable and has a big balcony from which I can see the mountain and the sea. I was conscious that I was extremely privileged in comparison to the majority of people in South Africa and Africa.

Still the sadness kept hovering.

A few days later I read an interview with David Kessler, who had worked with the famous Elizabeth Kübler-Ross on the five stages of grief. The penny dropped. I was grieving and so was the rest of the world.

We were grieving for our world that had changed. We were grieving because we feared economic uncertainty. We were grieving because people were dying and we didn't know if it would happen to us.

In the car after my scan, I thought about that time, now almost 24 months later. COVID was still part of our lives, perhaps even more. In March 2020 we thought that three weeks of strict quarantine might put an end to the pandemic. How wrong we were. Over the next two years, hundreds of millions of people had contracted the virus and millions had died. Despite vaccines being freely available (at least to those in the "developed" world), there seemed to be no reprieve.

Quite the opposite. South African scientists had just

identified a new variant of the COVID-19 virus which was later named as Omicron. To show its "appreciation", Europe, the USA and many other countries within hours announced bans on flights from six southern African countries. These measures, which smacked of prejudice and were devoid of all scientific evidence, had immediate and disastrous implications for the South African economy.

From the outcry on social media, it was clear that people could not cope with much more.

Thinking about all of this I suddenly realised that what I was going through after the hysterectomy – the fear, the pain, the loneliness and the grief – were what we all have had to grapple with during COVID. Since the start of the pandemic, in March 2020, we have been facing a collective struggle as humanity tried to redefine ourselves in a world that has been changed forever – in the same way that I was trying to redefine myself in a body that no longer felt familiar.

Pope Francis, in his book *Let Us Dream*, says that any crisis requires us to stop – or a period of "stoppage"[13] as he calls it. COVID literally stopped the whole world dead in its tracks overnight, as did my hysterectomy to me. Physically I couldn't move for a while without extreme pain, but the much bigger challenge was the emotional pain.

---

[13] Pope Francis. *Let us Dream*. Simon and Schuster, 2020. p.35

As Pope Francis put it: "... these moments generate a tension, a crisis that reveals what is in our hearts."

There was no question that my heart was breaking wide open.

Goodbye beloved Arch

As the year came to an end, I was looking forward to the six-month anniversary of the operation. It was Christmas time, and my son was in South Africa for two months with his lovely new partner. After having months of physiotherapy in a heated pool I was feeling stronger. So, I had also decided to build a pool in my front garden. After weeks of construction, it was finally finished, and I was enjoying my daily swim.

Since we had to cancel the previous Christmas on short notice because of further lockdowns, I was looking forward to a time of togetherness with family and friends.

Then the Omicron variant hit.

First, my sister in Johannesburg and her one son got infected. Then my mum was laid low. My other sister had seen my mum and helped her to do the rapid test (which showed a positive result) and then had to self-isolate as a precaution. My children had visited their 93-year-old grandmother on the Verwoerd side, who was so weak that my daughter insisted that she be hospitalized. It turned out that both she and their grandfather were infected.
So, my children had been exposed too.

Christmas was cancelled yet again. It was all starting to feel like too much.

The day after Christmas, while meditating, I got a call from a local radio station.

"Hi, Melanie. We were hoping you can go on air in the next few minutes and comment on the Tutu event," said the producer.

My heart sunk and a deep sense of gloom enveloped me.

"I haven't heard," I said, feeling my body starting to quiver. "Has he died?"

My mind immediately went back to a sunny day in Dublin around 2004.

At the time I was South Africa's Ambassador to Ireland and the Arch (as he was called) was in Dublin for a reconciliation event. During a press event he spotted a photographer's motorbike and asked if he could get on it. He got on and then chuckled:

"Spring op (jump on), let's give these guys something to talk about."

Of course, I did and the next day the photo of us on the motorbike was on the front pages of the many Irish newspapers.

I really loved the Arch and even though I would never be so arrogant as to describe us as being friends, my path crossed his at some of the most important milestones in my personal and political life.

The first time I met the Arch was during the late 1980s, at Stellenbosch University. It was his first visit to the university and, most probably, the first visit of any black speaker. For days, there were protests on campus against his appearance, and pamphlets were distributed using selective quotes to "prove" that he was "the antichrist" and "a communist".

On the evening of his appearance, tempers were fraying. The security police were everywhere, as were the bomb squad, military and campus police. It was not long before the handful of left-wing students got into physical fights inside the venue with the more mainstream students.

The Arch, however, came into the hall calmly and faced the angry crowd. "Goeie naand" (good evening), he said in Afrikaans. You could hear a pin drop and the discomfort among the majority of students was tangible. He then went on to tell a very funny joke about how he and Brigitte Bardot ended up together in heaven. His well-known high-pitched laughter disarmed even the most conservative in the audience, and by the end of the evening he had all of them eating out of the palm of his hand. He even got a standing ovation.

Though I had already started to question the political ideology that I had been taught since infancy, I knew that night for sure that my political path would lead me closer to Tutu and away from the Bothas and De Klerks of our time.

A few years later it was he who hugged me tightly on the day I was inaugurated as an MP for the ANC, reminding me to continue to be brave.

Two years later, he was the one who showed us again what

true courage was when he cried with us as our shameful past was exposed at the TRC (Truth and Reconciliation Commission).

When people so bravely exposed their almost unbearable pain and grief, he comforted them and held them – both physically and emotionally. And when the apartheid leaders failed to apologise, he, the one who had nothing to apologise for, apologised to victims, because someone had to.

Then, when I am sure he would have liked to take a rest after the decades of struggle and the gruelling TRC process, he had to become our voice of conscience yet again. As the morally corrupt decisions, abuses of power, and human rights abuses confronted us at a pace no one could have thought possible pre-1994, it was the Arch who fearlessly continued to speak out.

By this time, I was already in Ireland as Ambassador, and he came to stay a few times with me and my family. To this day, I try (rather unsuccessfully) to emulate his routine of early morning prayer and quiet time, which I observed him doing without fail every day.

Although a man of the cloth, part of the Arch's greatness was that he never took himself too seriously and, although deeply spiritual, he was not pious.

Once, when he stayed with me, Bono from U2 and his wife Ali came over to see the Arch. The Arch offered to say a prayer and to do a blessing for the about-to-be-released "How to Dismantle an Atomic Bomb" album. We stood in a circle as the Arch prayed in Xhosa first, and when it sounded like he was winding down, Bono, in a real rock 'n' roll gesture, lifted up his fist into the air and said "Amen!"

The Arch opened his one eye and said: "I am not finished, man!" He then closed his eyes and continued in Afrikaans . . . Once more, it sounded like he was winding down, but before Bono could do anything, the Arch, again with one eye closed, said: "Not yet!" He continued in English and then gave Bono a little nudge: "Now!" and Bono threw his fist into the air with an "Amen!"

A few years later I hosted an informal dinner for the Arch and a few friends in a private room of a restaurant in Dublin. We had a lovely evening. However, in the middle of a very intense and heated discussion about the peace process in Northern Island, the door to the private room suddenly swung open and two scantily dressed burlesque dancers came in.

A silence fell in the room and conscious that we were in the presence of a holy man, we stared over at them in horror. "Hello," the two women purred. Luckily, before any more could happen, a frazzled manager ran in. "Wrong room, wrong room," he said, "Your function is upstairs!" There was a slightly uncomfortable pause after they left, but then the Arch said with exaggerated "disappointment": "That was not very Christian to chase them out like that. We should invite them back for something to eat. They looked hungry."

His humour and lack of piousness did not mean that he wasn't faithful to his calling as spiritual leader. A few years ago, I was due to meet the Arch. His assistant called and said: "The Arch wants to know when you were last in church." I had to admit not too recently to which she said: "The Arch suspected that and says you must come to the Eucharist on Friday and then you can have coffee afterwards."

I did, of course.

He also never stopped "sweating the small stuff". During one of his visits in Dublin, he made my driver stop in a business area and told me to wait in the car while he got something. A few days later a big bunch of flowers arrived with a card: "Thank you for everything, ousie."

It felt to me that with the death of the Arch, South Africa and the whole world lost a spiritual giant, our unerring moral compass. For almost seven decades, when so many often felt unheard and unseen because of the colour of their skin or economic status, the Arch was always there.

Now he was no longer with us, and the media wanted to speak to me about him.

I was so heartbroken that I didn't know how I would do it. I agreed to do an interview with a friend of mine, who is a brilliant broadcaster and who I knew would handle it sensitively. John got me through the interview with gentleness and afterwards I had a good cry.

I then listened to Beethoven's piano concert no 1.

One of my fondest memories of the Arch is spending a few

hours interviewing him once. We sat on a couch in his hotel room and for most of the interview he had his arm around me. At some stage I asked him what his favourite piece of music was. To my great surprise he said: "Beethoven's piano concerto number 1." He then starting to hum it – with perfect pitch and timing.

That evening I went with my son and his partner to pay our respects at the cathedral. Next to St. Georges Cathedral there is a lovely wooden arch – built in his honour and named "the arch for the Arch". It had been illuminated in the deep purple of his liturgical garments. The City Hall and Table Mountain were also lit up with deep purple lights (his favourite colour), but also, appropriately, the colour of mourning.

The rest of the week I – and the rest of South Africa – were filled with the sadness and memories of the Arch. I was filled with anxiety and despair, as I wondered how the country would go forward now that the huge anchor that kept the South African ship from drifting into catastrophe was gone.

The Arch had planned his funeral meticulously. COVID restricted the number of people who could attend, so I joined the millions watching on TV while the bells of the cathedral, which is close to my house, rang their sad lament.

My heart felt warm as I saw the simple pine coffin with just a few carnations laid on it. He wanted none of the ostentatious drama of a state funeral. It was as intimate and humble as the funeral of a world-famous figure could be.

The next day someone sent me the photos of a tiny little pine box with his ashes being lowered into the floor of the Cathedral. Only his family was there – as he had wanted.

The evening of his funeral was New Year's Eve, and I was alone. I have always preferred it that way and have for years avoided parties – choosing instead to spend time in meditation and doing little rituals to say goodbye to the old year whilst setting intentions for the year to come.

That year, I sat outside in my garden next to my pool thinking of all the pain and loss of the past year. With my dog faithfully asleep next to me on the grass, I whispered:

"Hamba kahle, (walk well) dearest Arch. This ousie will miss you." Then I affirmed: "This has to be a better year."

I knew that I wanted to be clear about my vision for the upcoming year and decided to put some time aside for it.

But first there was another curve ball.

Fire!

The morning after the Arch's funeral, I woke up to the smell of smoke. Living on the slopes of Table Mountain we often have big mountain fires that force us to evacuate, but this time the smoke seemed to come from the opposite direction.

I looked at my phone to see if there were any alerts from the neighbourhood groups. There were none – just a text from my daughter.

When I opened it, I gasped.

She had sent me photos that her paramedic husband had got from his colleagues.

Parliament was burning.

In 1994, a few months after I was elected as a member of parliament, I had decided to move to Cape Town. The daily (sometimes twice daily) commute between Cape Town and Stellenbosch – 55 km away along the treacherous N2 highway – was becoming too tiring and stressful.

For weeks I had looked at houses close to parliament. My one precondition was that I wanted to be able to go home and feed my children when we were working evening sessions and still get into parliament within five minutes should there be an unexpected vote.

So, we looked and looked, but everything was too

expensive. One night, after a late session, I was starting my long journey home, when I saw a "for sale" board at the beginning of what was then De Waal Drive, now renamed Philip Skosana Drive. On the spur of the moment, I turned off into the new development.

It was dark, but I found an agent in a nearby sales office who took me to the open plots of land. With the lights of the city around me, I felt slightly dizzy and knew this was where I wanted to live. I knew too that my husband would take some convincing. We had built our previous house from scratch, and Wilhelm wasn't keen on the stress of building again, but I had instantly fallen in love with the area. Not only would we be living close to parliament, but it was affordable too!

A very stressful year followed, with me managing the building project, doing parliamentary and constituency work, finishing my Masters' degree – all with two children under the age of four.

Yet it was worth it.

I could see the house from my office window in parliament, which meant that I could see my children between committee meetings. At night I was able to feed and put them to bed, before rushing back to work. Importantly I could make it back in time to vote if necessary.

I had timed it down to the second. The bells would ring for five minutes before the doors of the chamber would be locked. So, after the call from my bench mates who kindly agreed to inform me if there was an unexpected vote, I would jump in my car, speed down the hill into the underground garage, up the lift and into my seat close to the door – just in time.

On more than one occasion the Speaker of the House would smile at me while shaking her head as I flew in through the door at the last minute.

I love my house and during my divorce I fought hard to keep it. Thankfully, Wilhelm never had the same love for it and agreed that I could keep it in exchange for other properties. I let it out while I lived in Ireland. After my return to South Africa and some renovations, it became my safe haven and happy space once more.

Now, standing on the balcony, I watched the dark black smoke spiralling up and the sounds of sirens filling the air as more and more fire engines rushed to the scene. This was clearly a big blaze.

It took two days for the fire to be extinguished, by which time, most of the majestic building had been destroyed.

I felt heartbroken.

My first visit to parliament had been during the Apartheid days and it nearly ended with Wilhelm and I being thrown out. I wish I could say that it was because of some political or activist action. It wasn't. We were invited to lunch by an old university friend of Wilhelm's who was an MP.

As we headed through the lobby of the old Assembly (the

former all-white parliament) towards the dining room, we were stopped by an usher.

"Sorry sir, you cannot go any further."

"Why?" we wanted to know.

"You need to wear a tie and jacket in Parliament," he said sternly, frowning disapprovingly at Wilhelm's student attire.

Luckily, they kept some spare jackets and ties, and we were finally allowed to enter the great big dining hall, where British Prime Minister Harold Macmillan had given his famous "Winds of Change" speech in 1960.

A few years later, we were showing some Australian friends around Cape Town. On the spur of the moment, we decided to see if we could show them parliament.

Wilhelm is the grandson of the former Prime Minister HF Verwoerd, who is generally regarded as the architect of Apartheid. Verwoerd's assassination in Parliament in 1966 was big news. The whites mourned his death, whilst black South African celebrated.

Our visit was still during Apartheid and on hearing Wilhelm's surname, the white policemen at the gate ushered us in and called someone to come and meet us. The lady was clearly very impressed to meet a Verwoerd grandson and led us into the Old Assembly chamber where Wilhelm's grandfather was assassinated.

To our guests' horror, she described the incident in great detail.

Turning to Wilhelm, she said: "I don't know what you heard, but I was told that Tsafendas (the assassin) had to stab him quite a few times."

She then pointed out a faint brown stain on the carpet.

"That is still from the blood," she said. "They could never completely get it out."

My daughter, who was less than a year old, was getting restless and needed to be fed. So, while our guide was continuing her shock and horror commentary, I popped into one of the benches and fed her under my shirt.

When it was time to move on, she was not done and protested loudly.

An old hand at breastfeeding by then, I popped her back on, pulled my top as low as possible, and followed the guide through the maze of parliamentary passages.

Little did I know that less than four years later I would be back, but this time as an elected MP for the ANC – the party that Verwoerd had banned and whose leader, Nelson Mandela, he had incarcerated.

A few days after the 1994 election, the ANC held their first caucus meeting in the same Old Assembly Chamber and the irony of the moment was not lost upon us. This time, the lobby was alive with noise, children were running around, and people loudly and happily greeted each other. Ties and jackets were nowhere to be seen, as most people had dressed in traditional outfits.

In the caucus room, I craned my neck. The stain was still there, but now, sitting at the bench where Verwoerd had died, sat Nelson Mandela. I realised that Madiba was looking at me across the floor. Our eyes locked and for a brief moment he held my gaze. He smiled and nodded at me. Emotions were starting to overwhelm me, and I was not the only one.

Thabo Mbeki, who would five years later become President, was chairing the meeting and as was the practice, we were asked to stand for the national anthem. More than two hundred people rose to their feet and lifted their fists into the air. There was a moment of silence and then, spontaneously, a woman started "Nkosi Sikelele Afrika" - God Bless Africa. Slowly the sea of 250 voices filled the hall. It was as if these activists and freedom fighters, through their voices, and through their prayer, wanted to cleanse the place.

And so, they did.

Parliament was transformed after 1994. The buildings remained fundamentally the same, but everything else changed. Of course, the elected members now reflected the wishes of the majority. The staff represented of the demographics of the country. The art and even the menus changed to celebrate our glorious diversity. It was no longer a place intended to keep the populace out, but welcomed people in. It had become a people's parliament.

Anyone who has ever served there will tell you that it is a special place. When in session, MPs spend almost all their waking hours there. It becomes your home and your colleagues become your family – albeit, like most families, a rather dysfunctional one.

In the mornings you would greet everyone you would come across and ask if they were well and had a good night. In the evenings you would say good night. In between, you had breakfast, lunch and often dinner together and of course the drinkers would share some time in the pub as well. Your colleagues were the ones with whom you shared your stress, exhaustion, frustrations and worries, because only they understood the strain of being an elected representative. And you laughed, you laughed a lot, not only because of the absurdity of each day's political theatre, but because it kept you sane.

Our parliament in Cape Town was a living and breathing space. It was one of the few places other than museums that reminded us of where we had come from and could never return to, whilst also celebrating what we had overcome and could become.

Places matter because people are shaped not only by ideas, but by the spaces that surround them, and parliament was such a place and more - it was a symbol of the power of people to do good and overcome evil.

One night, as the embers were still smouldering in what was left of the beautiful buildings, I realised that it had been a year of fire for me. It had started on my birthday. Early on the 18th of April there were reports of a small fire on Table Mountain. This was nothing new but fanned by very strong winds it grew and spread fast. By the evening all the people living in my road stood outside watching as the sky turned orange – a sign that the flames were getting close. Someone suddenly remembered that it was my birthday and ran inside to get some wine. The fire fighters joined in – flashing their lights – while everyone sang happy birthday. The next morning, we had to evacuate as trees in the park behind us exploded in massive fire balls. Luckily the wind turned just meters before the fire reached our houses.

Two months later, as I woke up from anaesthetic, I watched in horror on nearby TV screens the reports of people looting and setting places alight. Former president Zuma had been found guilty on contempt of court charges and sentenced to 15 months in prison. After a stand-off he eventually handed himself over to the police, but some of his supporters started to cause mayhem which quickly spread to other parts of the country.

Over the next few days, thousands of shops were burnt or looted. People lost their lives, and billions were lost to the economy. In a morphine haze, I couldn't help thinking about how, at the same time as I was walking through fire with my body, my beloved country was going up in smoke.

Now, as the year ended, my beloved parliament was also lying in ashes. So much destruction – so much pain. Yet, as much as fire represented destruction and death, it could also be the beginning of rebirth or resurrection. The natural habitat on Table Mountain, where I live, actually needs a fire every few years in order for the seeds to germinate.

Looking out at the smoke still rising in the distance, I prayed silently: "Please, let this be the beginning of some rebirth for parliament, our country and... me. Let it be a year of new beginnings."

Finding my vision

A few days after New Year, I took part in a vision board workshop facilitated by a wonderful Jamaican woman named Nadine McNeil.

I had met Nadine 18 months earlier during a visit to Bali. After a few days in a silent retreat, I checked into the Yoga Barn centre in a town called Ubud. I'm not a massive fan of Ubud. After Elizabeth Gilbert's *Eat Pray Love* book, the place became even more popular with foreign tourists and expats, and it felt very inauthentic to me.

Still, I wanted to do an Ayurvedic course which was taking place in Ubud. Scanning through the seemingly endless array of classes and workshops offered at Yoga Barn, my eyes caught a Women's Circle workshop. I immediately felt drawn to it.

However, as the time drew closer, I wasn't so keen. It was boiling hot, I was tired and dreaded the idea of being in a room full of people. Yet, there was this strong urge to go. I was the first to arrive and waited outside the venue. Just as I considered leaving, a stunning Jamaican woman in a see-through white, flowing dress with the strongest energy I have ever experienced came outside and told me to please wait since we would start soon. So, I did.

It was Nadine, who would be facilitating the workshop. The next few hours would be life altering and saving. After we discovered that we had both worked for UNICEF,

Nadine and I connected almost immediately and over the next few months our friendship would blossom.

When COVID hit, Nadine hosted Women's Circles that would become instrumental in my healing. This group of exceptional and deeply compassionate women "met" every week via Zoom. We supported each other as work disappeared, families separated, and the emotional strain of isolation took its toll. These circles continue to this day and even though new women join frequently, the core group of women, who have been there since early 2020, remains. We have become soul mates over thousands of miles.

At the beginning of 2022, Nadine advertised a vision board workshop on Zoom. I had done a number of vision boards or collages of my goals and visions before, yet I felt drawn to enrol. The problem was that since Nadine had to accommodate various time zones around the globe mine would only start at nine pm.

"Don't worry, you will be so inspired you won't even feel the time," Nadine assured me.

In the week leading up to the workshop I bought art supplies and started to think how I wanted my board to look. I wanted it to be beautiful and to inspire me. Also, I didn't want it to be in my usual square, organized, neat pattern. I was no longer the woman of the years gone by – and my board needed to reflect that. So, I played around with ideas of circles and the feminine figure, but nothing felt right, so I postponed the final decision to the evening of the workshop.

After an initial meditation, Nadine gave us some guidance. Then (I forget now in what context), she mentioned a lotus flower. Something in me shifted.

I knew intuitively that the image of the lotus flower was what I needed to guide me through the next few months.

A few years ago, I had watched an episode of "Chef's Table" on Netflix. The episode focuses on a Korean Buddhist monk, Jeong Kwan, and at some point in the episode, she makes lotus tea. It is one of my favourite television moments ever. Jeong Kwan gently takes a lotus flower and places it in a bowl of water. Then with chopsticks, she slowly and gently opens every leaf, taking her time in order not to damage the fragile petals. Every time I watch this, I am mesmerised. Her state of complete calm and mindfulness combined with the fragility of the lotus flower moves me deeply.

With roots in the mud, lotus flowers disappear every night into the water only to reappear in the morning to bloom again. In many cultures this extraordinary flower is regarded as a symbol of rebirth and spiritual growth, which could not be more appropriate for what I was going through.

I had no doubt that I was on a journey of intense growth and rebirth, kickstarted by the operation. After all, how could I go back to my old life, when my soul and body felt totally different?

I had no idea where it would end up. In fact, I was not even clear where I wanted the journey to end up. All I knew was that, like any birth, there was a point after which it could not be stopped and I had passed that point.

I was also due a change. I had a few weeks earlier come to the realisation that my life ran in seven-year cycles.

I started school in 1973. Seven years later, in 1980, we moved to another town where I started high school. Seven years after that I got married. In 1994, seven years after my marriage, I was elected as a member of parliament. After seven years in parliament, I was appointed an ambassador in 2001. I would meet Gerry seven years later after my marriage with Wilhelm ended 21 years after we first met. I would leave Ireland seven years after Gerry and I started our relationship and his subsequent death. Returning to South Africa I had re-invented myself as a political analyst and it was now seven years later.

I knew that some kind of change was inevitable.

Interestingly enough, I would later read that the number seven represents completeness. How appropriate.

Back at the vision board workshop, I knew that a year was too long to work with. I could and wanted to only post on the board my vision for the next six months. Especially since I had just had a session with two people that had become important in my life.

Fifteen years earlier, during the last months of my failing marriage, my Irish friend Brid gifted me a session with an astrologer in Dublin. I was sceptical and decided not to give anything away during the reading. Yet, after just a few minutes with Andrew Smith, I was flabbergasted. He mentioned certain events that he could have found on the internet, but the accuracy of certain dates and events in my past which had not been recorded anywhere was astonishing.

Given that the oceans' tides and women's cycles are determined by the moon, it made sense to me that we are also more generally impacted by the planets. Andrew is also not one for cheap predictions and doomsday scenarios, so over the years I have asked his help when I've felt stuck or lost. He is always reassuring and his insights helpful.

Five months after my operation, I felt like I had hit a wall. The physical healing was fine, but mentally I was still struggling to come to terms with everything. Work felt tedious and mundane, and I wanted nothing more than to withdraw to think and write. It freaked me out. What if I never wanted to go back to work again? What about money? How would I survive?

Andrew kindly squeezed me in.

As luck would have it, I had also experienced a session the week before with an amazing woman I had met during my first trip to Bali. At the retreat place, one of the optional extras was a tarot card reading. I was dubious. I had seen too many movies and really didn't want some scammer telling me that I was going to marry a prince – or die soon. Yet, the very level-headed women running the retreat couldn't stop speaking about Szilvia Galambos and how helpful she had been to sort out particularly deep-seated emotional problems.

I became intrigued and decided to "risk" it. I loved Szilvia from the moment I met her. Kindness radiated from her, and she clearly had a gift. I don't understand how tarot or other cards work, but I know that in the right hands, they can be very helpful and accurate. I have come to accept that some people who are exceptionally intuitive can use these cards to heal others and lighten their burdens.

The extraordinary thing was that both Andrew in Ireland and Szilvia in Bali came up with exactly the same advice.

I needed silence. I needed to be, (as Andrew put it), "in my lady cave" in order to take stock, dream and figure out what I was doing next in my life. For at least the next six months it was crucial that I focused on me. I needed to recovery physically and mentally, reconnect with my spiritual self, shed what no longer served me and write!

As scary as that was, I knew I had no choice. I had already withdrawn to some extent by saying "no" to many things, but it felt like I had to do more and be more aware and intentional about it.

After midnight I stepped back to look at my completed vision board.

It was in the shape of a lotus flower with four big leaves and two small ones.

At the centre I had written the words "silence" and

"retreat". Each leaf held my commitments to myself. I would focus on my body, I would deepen my spiritual practice, I would have my voice heard and I would shed whatever was holding me back.

I also added two smaller leaves with the words "travel" and "beauty" on them.

It seemed to me that this vision would be the roadmap that would lead me to both physical and emotional healing. Most importantly, I was hoping that it would help me to find an answer to the most important questions: What were my deepest desires and what gave me joy?

Saying no

"Do you think I have done enough with my life?" I asked Gerry a few months before he died.

He focussed intensely on me, as only he could.

"Yes! In terms of achievements and other people you have done more than enough," he said after a few seconds.

"In terms of you, you are only starting."

That conversation has always stayed with me and now more than ten years later, it felt that I had to heed his words. I had to focus on me. This meant that I had to learn to say "No" – something I – like most women – find almost impossible to do.

Shonda Rhimes wrote a fantastic book called *Year of Yes*. Boy, can this creator and writer of the TV shows "Grey's Anatomy", "Scandal" and "Private Practice" write! In it she describes how, despite being super successful, she tended to avoid social events, press interviews, media appearances etc. The turning point came when her sister Delorse remarked one day: "You never say yes to anything. At that point Shonda decided to say yes – for a year.

The book touched me. I knew that place of saying no. Like Shonda, I am an introvert who had to learn how to function and survive whilst having a very public life, albeit it not on the Shonda Rhimes level.

I learnt how to do it (say yes) and I was good at it, but it took a toll physical and emotionally. So, in order to recover from the "overheating" of social and work life, I would crave quiet home time. Dinner and cocktail parties were work – and it was hard work.

Over the years, I would tie myself into knots trying to avoid invitations to parties and finding excuses for other social invites. So, I wondered if there was something in Shonda's book that I could emulate?

Clearly there were some valuable lessons in it, but they didn't really resonate with me. I read the book a second time, thinking I had missed something. I enjoyed it as much, if not more, but still felt that it wasn't what my soul wanted or needed.

As the post-operative nudge to live life differently and the need to find time for silence and withdrawal became more pressing, I knew that I had to go through a phase of saying no. It had been necessary to remove some organs that were threatening my wellness. Now, it seemed I had to shed that which was no longer serving me so that I could live a life of wholeness – perhaps for the first time.

To allow that journey to unfold I needed to carve out time to be able to think and write. This meant saying no to some of my work engagements – something that would almost paralyse me with fear.

After almost 12 years in Ireland, I had very few connections left in South Africa on my return and my public profile was non-existent. I came home to no work and no income. It took ten hard years to create a viable business as a political analyst.

My youngest sister had kindly allowed me to stay in her Cape Town apartment for free for a year. I applied for endless jobs in the NGO and development sector, but it quickly became obvious that a very public battle with UNICEF Ireland – who had fired me after Gerry died because of what they called the "ongoing media attention surrounding his death" – had closed those doors for me.

I debated going back into active politics, but the principled ANC of Nelson Mandela was fast decaying into a party of corruption and patronage, and I no longer felt at home there.

I published two books, but as is true of most books, they brought in about two months' coffee money.

It was a dark and challenging time.

The breakthrough came after reconnecting with the late well-known author and political analyst, Allister Sparks. With his encouragement I started to do political analysis.

The relief of doing something I enjoyed – and being paid for it – was indescribable. I said yes to everything I was asked to do. As my profile grew, so did the requests. I would be away from home 100 nights in a year, often handling up to four paid speaking engagements per day.

Of course, I still supported my children, was there for family and friends, looked after my pets and tried to run a perfect household. Inevitably, I became totally burnt out. Still, I kept saying yes. The memory of no job and no money as well as my innate drive towards success made it impossible to say no.

At the end of one particularly gruelling year, I was asked to stand in for a top radio host during the December period. I was scared out of my mind at the prospect of doing the daily three-hour drive time show, but I didn't know how to say no.

So, I said yes.

It nearly killed me.

Unless you have done it, it is impossible to understand how stressful daily live radio or TV broadcasting is – especially if you are a perfectionist and like to be in control. The unpredictability, the relentless pace and the fact that you can never have "dead air", demands a special type of resilience.

After the three weeks I was at the point of collapse.

One day sitting at the hairdressers, I was paging through a women's magazine. I would usually take a book or work, but on this day I was so tired I couldn't muster up the energy to read.

As I paged bleary eyed through the magazine, I suddenly saw an article about a women's retreat in Bali. I looked closer. It sounded amazing, but going halfway around the world to have a holiday on my own? Could I do that? And it wasn't cheap.

I counted the years since I had last taken a holiday.

Eight!

It had been eight years since Gerry and I had travelled to South Africa for three weeks on a glorious holiday a year before catastrophe hit. Shockingly, it was the last time I had taken a break.

I took a photo of the article on my phone and had a quick look at my bank account.

Back home I looked up flights and then emailed the retreat place. "I know this is short notice, but can I perhaps come in a few days' time?"

The next morning when I woke up the answer was there. "We have one more space left. Come! We would love to have you." Before I could talk myself out of it, I booked the flights and sent the deposit.

Later that day, my kids were watching TV. "Hey, I'm going to Bali next week," I said casually. They both nodded absently and continued watching TV.

I waited for it to sink in.

Five, four, three...

I watched as they suddenly looked at one another.

"What?" said my daughter.

"I decided to go to Bali for a holiday."

"With whom?" they said in unison.

"No one, just me."

There was a long pause as they both stared at me.

"Are you having some mid-life crisis?" asked my son.

"Nope, I'm just having a holiday for my 50th birthday."

Years later I would read in one of Sue Monk Kidd's books that women often take life changing journeys in the year that they turn fifty.

Bali was that for me. I would return four times in the next five years.

On the first trip, I met a fantastic healer and guide, Malcolm Nicolls. Malcolm was the first one to teach me the importance of saying no. Over the years, he would gently nudge me to say no to what I didn't want to do, in order to make space for what I really did want to do.

That sounds simple, but it was extremely difficult for me – as I'm sure it is for most women. I hate disappointing people and I have a belief that I can always keep going. Then there is the fear of becoming a bag lady – that I would run out of money.

So, saying no – especially to work requests – seemed impossible.

Malcolm suggested that I start with taking Fridays off. I was my own boss, so why not schedule that day for myself? I nearly passed out at the thought of it. Yet, I craved it.

I gradually started to tell people that I was fully booked on Fridays. The problem was that I then over-booked my other days.

Yet, I treasured Fridays.

Then the COVID pandemic hit. With public meetings no longer possible, work slowed down significantly as did my income, so again I would take anything I could do via Zoom.

After the operation, I took a few weeks to recuperate. Then I started to say yes to everything again. After all, the world was still deeply in the COVID depression, so how on earth could I say no to work opportunities, in order to have time for introspection and writing?

The problem was that I got more and more frustrated and unhappy. I started to resent the work that was keeping me away from what my soul was calling for. It also felt as if my physical and mental healing had slowed: physical pain returned, and my dreams were filled with dark nightmares.

After a few more discussions with Malcolm, I knew I had

no choice. My work was of course my only source of income, but in future I would only say yes to the projects that paid well. Anything else, I would decline politely.

It would be my year of No.

I needed to say No, in order to say Yes,

That meant saying no to the significant number of media requests I got on a weekly basis. I explained that I needed time to fully heal – which, to my surprise, almost all the journalists understood and empathised with.

Yet, every time I said no, I felt physically sick. Profile is important in the business I'm in and with more and more analysts coming onto the scene I knew it was very risky.

Yet, after the initial feeling of panic, I would feel an enormous sense of relief in my body and soul – at least until my mind stepped in with doomsday scenarios. I knew I had to trust that I was doing the right thing – and that it was not a permanent decision. I had to trust that if I wanted to, I could ramp it up again.

Of course, there were also family demands. Thankfully, my kids were now grown and for the first time in three decades I no longer had any of them on my credit cards (so to speak). Both had good jobs and seemed happy and settled in their lives. This created a sense of freedom after two decades of being responsible for their financial, emotional and physical wellbeing.

During this time my daughter confided to me that she

wanted to get pregnant. I was delighted for her. I knew that she had always wanted to have children and the idea of having a little person in our lives truly excited me. I had even been buying children's books – mostly with feminist story lines – for years, in anticipation of grandchildren. I also had a whole bag full of little baby outfits.

Still, I was worried about her, because she had suffered from Lyme disease which had gone undiagnosed for almost ten years. I also knew that once the baby was there, a new phase of secondary mothering would start again for me.

As much as I was looking forward to that, I was also desperate for some time just for me. That now seemed more urgent than ever. Assuming my daughter got pregnant easily, I had less than a year.

As the urgency in me grew, I gradually came to the realisation that this road I was on needed to be walked alone. There was no space or emotional energy for taking someone along for the ride. This was a solo journey that would require my full attention – which meant that I had to make some painful choices.

Walking it alone.

What makes memories and trauma so potent?

A few months after the operation, I suddenly started to feel very anxious. I have never experienced a panic attack, but on more than one occasion I've known that I was on the edge of one.

I had been feeling a lot better, so I didn't understand what was going on.

After a lot of soul searching I realized that I was having PTSD symptoms again. More soul searching followed, together with careful interrogation of what preceded every episode. Eventually the penny dropped.

About seven months before the operation, I had reconnected with an old acquaintance. We had actually met up 18 months before that and had considered the possibility of a relationship, but there were obstacles and eventually nothing came of it.

A year and a half later we reconnected and this time we became close. He was smitten with me, and I was flattered and really liked him, but the voice deep inside me whispered warnings. Conscious of my tendency to talk myself out of relationships before even giving them a try, I ignored the voice.

He was kind, gentle and extremely supportive – especially in the time prior to the operation. When I went to see the surgeon, he held my hand and took me to the hospital on the day of the operation.

However, when I came home a few days after the operation, I didn't want him close to me. It was just too intimate, too messy. I needed women to soothe me, look after me and to sit with my shock and pain.

A few weeks later, I was happy to recuperate at his house but the warning voice inside me was becoming louder.

Eventually, I realized that I needed space to figure out who I was after the operation. He agreed but we still saw and spoke to each other daily.

Having been separated for years, he was in the final stages of his divorce. One of the agreements was that he and his wife would retain one property collectively, with equal rights to the use of it.

Under most circumstances that would be fine, except that the property in question was the one he and I were living in at that time.

"Where would I go, when she comes to visit?" I asked when he first raised it with me.

"You can stay," he responded, to my utter surprise. It was clear to me that this would never work. One of us would feel like an outsider and since this was her house – it was not going to be her.

Despite my gentle nudging, he did nothing about my

concern and as Christmas approached she informed him that she wanted the family to have time together in the Cape Town house.

And just like that – the PTSD was back.

The ex-who-is-not-quite-an-ex was a repeat of what I had gone through with Gerry a decade previously. He had been separated for years by the time we started to see each other but Irish divorce law at that time required couples to be separated for at least four years before a formal separation would be granted

Gerry died three short weeks before the four years were over.

Even though he and I had lived together and shared every aspect of our lives, his ex-wife was very present, and this became unbearable after his death. I was immediately informed that I had no standing in law and was instructed to remove my possessions from the house we shared.

Despite having been the one who found him on our bedroom floor on the day of his death, I had to get permission from his wife to see his body afterwards. She brought his body back to the house they had shared when they were married and held a wake for him there. I was not invited. At the funeral she was the one who spoke and at the grave she took centre stage.

Together with the pain of losing Gerry, this denial made life almost unbearable at the time.

I had thought that I had made peace with all of that, yet more than a decade later, the arrival of my new partner's wife triggered deep and dark memories. To the point that I felt physically sick and unable to fully function.

I was taken aback by all of this.

I had spent a lot of time during the previous decade coming to terms with the trauma of Gerry's death and had reached a place where I felt I was free of the worst of it. Yet, it now became clear that I had not dealt with the secondary trauma caused by the events after his death.

I gradually came to grips with what had happened to me.

In the weeks and months after Gerry died, my feelings, my pain, my grief and even my existence had been denied. For months I was portrayed by the media as the "other woman" or even worse, my existence as Gerry's partner was just ignored.

Now, years later, while this new relationship would be of little or no interest to the media, the scars of the past were too deep. I knew that I could never put myself into a position of the "other woman" again.

So, I ended the relationship.

As the weeks went on, I realised that even beyond the traumas around Gerry's death, and the painful decision I had just made, yet another enormous issue loomed: I had started to ask myself a deeper, far more fundamental question.

Why have a relationship at all?

Of course, I understood that a relationship is often important for women when they want to have children. It had been for me, partly because cultural and religious norms dictated it, but also because I knew that single motherhood is extremely hard work.

I also understood that when two people have been together for many decades a sense of "zein und zeit"- a comfort and familiarity with the togetherness of many decades – can grow between them. Even if – as often happens – important elements of their love have died, they will choose to stay together because of the comfort familiarity brings.

Of course, many women are financially trapped, and can't escape their marriage even if they want to. In my case however, I have had my children, I don't want to, nor can I have any more. I have never had anyone support me financially. I like my own company. Despite being alone most of the time – I'm not lonely.

I am fine on my own.

So why would I want a relationship? Why risk it again?

With Gerry I had found real love. For the first time I wanted to be with someone all the time. I wanted to be inside his head, share his body and his life. Although it wasn't without challenges, it was the best time of my life.

The two years I was with him, I knew who I was meant to

be. I had found, in the words of Glennon Doyle, my wild again[14]. I felt safe and protected. I had his back and he had mine. For a short while the world became a safe place.

Then he died…

His death left me totally devastated and unravelled. Was I willing to go through that again?

The majority of single men are older than me and since men tend to die younger than women, the chance of my enduring another painful mourning process was very high.

Relationships also take up enormous amounts of time and energy. Was I willing to invest that again?

I got married when I was 20 years old. I had my first baby shortly after my 23rd birthday and my second two years later. I was elected as a member of parliament a few days after my 27th birthday and became an Ambassador at the age of 34. I got divorced at the age of 40.

During those two decades my life was totally absorbed with raising two children, the political struggle in South Africa and a calling to serve my country and Africa. I also tried – unsuccessfully – to keep a marriage together.

After my divorce, as the children's significant financial needs became mine to carry, I had at times struggled to keep my head above water.

---

[14] Glennon Doyle. *Untamed*. The Dial Press, 2020.

So, for more than 30 years I spent very little time, energy or money on me. That only started to change when I went to Bali for my 50th birthday and even then, it took a couple more years before my children were financially independent.

So now there was suddenly a freedom, a glorious freedom to focus on me.

Did I really want to fill that space with a man?

In her book *The Wisdom of Menopause*, Christiane Northrup notes that it is crucial for women to have a good hard look at all aspects of their relationships "for the sake of being true to yourself and protecting your emotional and physical health in the second part of your life." [15]

When reaching menopause, women are often for the first time free of the demands of raising children. At the same time, they also have a growing awareness of the inevitability of running out of time. So there is an urgency about following their hearts and deepest desires.

That was certainly true for me, and it became increasingly urgent after the operation. However, I had also struggled for a while with the question as to whether women in romantic relationships can ever truly be free.
When I would put that question to friends they would say: "Yes, if it is the right person."

Of course, that makes it easier. However, given that even

---

[15] Wisdom of menopause, Bantam Books, 2012

the most liberal societies still have significant remnants of patriarchy, it has always been clear to me that women in heterosexual relationships – either through direct demands or through subconscious beliefs – sacrifice their needs, energy and time far too often in order to keep their partners happy.

This has certainly been my experience with relationships over many years – all of which ended when I could no longer compromise who I wanted to be – a powerful, independent woman.

So, as I committed to my journey of healing and seeking freedom, I knew that this was a path I had to walk alone. If I wanted to give myself the time and space to truly dive deep, I had to be free of the complexities of relationships for a while.

I first needed to figure out who I now was, so that I could fully belong to myself.   That – and only that – is true freedom.

Only then will I be able to say in the words of Brené Brown:

"I know who I am; I'm clear about that, I am not going to negotiate who I am with you. Because then, I might fit in for you, but I no longer belong to myself. And that is a betrayal I am no longer willing to do."

In order to "show up" to the world and relationships again, I first had to find myself and that required a solo journey. I knew there would be no other way. It excited me, but also scared me. Yet, as Brené also said, very little that we ever do of value doesn't scare us shitless.

So, sitting in my garden late one night, I promised myself to shut myself off from any romantic relationship for the foreseeable future. As I watched the full moon rising over Cape Town, with Table Mountain in the background, I sighed a deep sigh of relief and whispered to myself:

"I am ok... I will be ok."

Crossing borders

"If you could do anything now, what would it be?" asked Malcolm on an early morning call in February.

As the year progressed, I started to feel extreme exhaustion. I knew it wasn't primarily physical, since I had just had a holiday. My body was still sore at times and my stomach had formed a floppy pouch around the scar, but I knew it wasn't that.

It was something deeper, that demanded attention.

Now, I listened in surprise as the words: "I would like to take a six-month sabbatical," fell out of my mouth.

"Where did that come from?" I wondered silently.

"There you go," said Malcolm. "How does it make you feel to say those words?'

I thought about it. I felt an immediate and enormous sense of relief. It was as if I could hear my soul applauding.

"A little scary, but also exciting," I said.

"Hold on to that feeling and figure out what you want to do with that time."

I immediately knew I wanted – needed – to travel.

I had not left Cape Town since March of 2020, when we got

Covid and the world came to a standstill. In some ways it suited me. Like many introverts, I enjoyed the quiet, slower pace of life. Still, it had now been almost two years and it felt like my soul was being suffocated.

I love South Africa, but having lived in Europe, I am always painfully aware of the fact that we really are on the most southern point of Africa. This makes traveling to Europe, Asia or America very time consuming and expensive. Living in South Africa is also exhausting. It takes a certain resilience to deal with the harsh climate, high level of crime, electricity blackouts and daily political intrigues.

So travel – if you can afford it – is like a breath of cool air.

I also immediately sensed that a physical journey would be instrumental for my inner journey. I literally needed to cross borders and physically fly away in order to cross the borders in my soul and learn how to fly again.

As Sue Monk-Kidd put it, I knew that crossing borders would allow me to cross into new and unknown regions of my soul.[16]

That evening I looked at my vision board. The small petal with "travel" written on it was still there. It had been a bit of an afterthought at the time, but now I knew that a physical journey was going to take centre stage in my emotional and spiritual journey.

That night I went back to Sue Monk-Kidd's book *Traveling*

---

[16] Ann Kidd Taylor and Sue Monk-Kidd. *Traveling with Pomegranates*. Viking, 2009, p.8

with Pomegranates, where she talks about crossing boundaries. "Is there an odyssey the female soul longs to make... one that has been blurred and lost within a culture awesomely alienated from the soul? If so, what sort of journey would it be?" she asked.[17]

Yes! I knew that travelling would be good for my physical healing, but most of all it was a calling from my soul.

As I fell asleep, I knew that the only question remaining unanswered was what type of journey it would be? Whatever it was, I knew intuitively that it would be part of the journey that had started six months before with the hysterectomy. A journey that insisted that I look at the dark, dusty corners of my psyche and soul in the hope of finding the freedom that I had wanted for as long as I could remember.

[17] Ann Kidd Taylor and Sue Monk-Kidd. *Traveling with Pomegranates.* Viking, 2009, p.6

Burying the bag lady

"How could I afford that?"

I could hear Malcolm smile over the thousands of miles that separated me from him in New Zealand. He knows me well and knew what was coming.

After blurting out that I wanted a sabbatical, I felt an initial sense of relief and excitement. It was quickly transformed into panic.

I have never quite been able to get rid of my "bag lady-fear". Over the years, I had tried to get to grips with it by understanding my money story (as Kate Northrup calls it)[18].

I grew up in the Calvinist tradition. This meant that hard work was deemed virtuous and idleness was never allowed. As a child I was often reminded that "idle hands are the devil's workshop" so to this day, I find it hard to watch television without also doing something with my hands – just in case the devil is lurking somewhere.

While hard work was seen as virtuous, money – and wealth in particular – bordered on the ungodly. As Max Weber's *Die Protestantische Ethik und der Geist des Kapitalismus* pointed out, religions like Calvinism forbade

---

[18] Kate Northrup. *Money: A Love Story: Untangle your financial woes and create the life you really want*. Hay House. 2013

the wasteful use of money – even if earned through hard work. Buying luxuries was regarded as sinful.

What constituted "waste" or "luxuries" was not clear to me, so I grew up with a general distrust in rich people and especially those who were "flashing it", as the Irish would say.

For all of my life, my mum would talk of her embarrassment at my biological dad's fondness for nice cars and other possessions. She would tell me how she would slide down in the seat of the car in parking lots, so that people would not see her in it. To me that sent a clear message: Money was at best problematic, at worst, dirty and dangerous.

After her second marriage, both she and my stepdad worked at the University of Stellenbosch and earned good salaries, so we lived comfortably, especially compared to the majority of people in the country. Still, I grew up with an awareness that "money did not grow on trees" and that it was important to be frugal. Sales were where we shopped for clothes and food shopping was done in bulk. Tea bags were re-used and wastage was not tolerated.

Although many of these lessons stood me in good stead later in my life when I would indeed not have a lot of money, there was always an underlying fear that money could run out at any time.

My upbringing and faith also taught me that money had to be earned through hard – very hard – work in order to be deserved. Otherwise, it could easily be "taken away". So, I worked extremely hard and as the years went on earned enough to live comfortably.

However, the fear of running out of money remained a continuous presence.

Money also became a big bone of contention in my marriage. Wilhelm and I got married while we were both students. After our stint in Oxford where we lived very frugally on his Rhodes scholarship, Wilhelm got a position as a junior lecturer at the University of Stellenbosch. The pay was really dreadful, so I started taking on part-time work, which also paid abysmally.

The money remained very tight, until I became a Member of Parliament, when my salary finally gave us a bit more breathing space, and when I became ambassador a few years later we lived a good life. Through careful management I was able to significantly reduce the mortgage on our house in South Africa.

As my term of office came to an end, the issue of money added strain to our already fragile marriage. Wilhelm wanted me to stop working for a while to spend time with the family. After eight gruelling years in politics and four in diplomacy, I was exhausted, so I was keen to take a break, but wanted to know where the money would come from.

Wilhelm's solution was to downscale dramatically. In principle I supported a "simple lifestyle", but I wasn't willing to move my children out of their schools – nor was

I happy to move to a working-class area in Belfast, which was one of his suggestions.

Stalemate.

Our different attitude to money wasn't the sole or even main reason for our separation, but it certainly played a big role.

Like most divorces, ours became acrimonious when it came to the financial settlement. I know we have different versions of the story, but in the end, I ended up paying for virtually all of the children's expenses for almost 15 years.

This left me petrified – especially since I was out of a job and therefore a salary. As is often the case with high earning women, I had left the managing of the money to Wilhelm during our marriage, partly to soothe his ego, but also because I had bought into the patriarchal belief that men knew more about money than women.

Like many before me, I came to the shocking realisation that this was far from the truth, so at the age of forty, I had to start from scratch learning the basics about money. It was frightening, but also empowering.

I read books and asked advice. Most importantly, I vowed that I would never be in that situation again. I had not expected a man to look after me, but now I promised myself to never be with a man who did not earn at least as much as me.

Ironically, towards the end of my relationship with Gerry,

I again ended up supporting a man. He earned a huge salary, but all (and more) went into sustaining his family. I felt that I had to step in.

Over the years I managed to earn enough money to keep me and my children comfortable. It was scary, hard work, but I did it. Yet, instead of feeling empowered, I remained fearful. "What if...?" was forever present.

It got a bit easier when my children became less dependent on me. My trip to Bali in the year I turned fifty was the first time I had incurred any big expense just for myself. After that trip I felt a bit more free to spend money on myself, including three more trips to Bali. Yet there was a consistent background hum of fear and scarcity.

I found it hard to understand. I had read so many books and done so much work on myself, why could I not rid myself of these deep fears?

A few nights before my discussion with Malcolm, I had woken up with the thought that I should make an inventory of all my money and debts. I did that from time to time – usually at the beginning of every year and every few months when I started to panic that money was running out. I put the light on, reached for my diary and did the calculations in the form of a lotus flower. When I was done, I looked at it. It wasn't that scary. My income had reduced significantly during COVID, but so had my expenses.

I had two mortgages, but they were manageable and thankfully I had no other debt. Before I fell asleep again, I wrote at the top of the page: "I have no idea why I had to do this, but here it is."

A few days later - after my "I need a six-month sabbatical "blurt to Malcolm, I opened my diary and looked at my abundance lotus flower. "Could I do this?"

My anxiety immediately rose again. I took a breath and looked up from my calculations.

On the desk in front of me was a small photograph that my mum had sent me the previous evening. It was of my maternal great-grandmother. It was the first time I had seen a photograph of her.

I picked it up and looked closely at the slightly faded picture. From our family tree, I knew that her name was Helena Johanna Jacoba Louw. She was born in 1883 and died in 1938. She was only 55 – my age – when she died. In the photographs, she was seated next to my great-grandfather, who looked serious – almost stern – dressed in a dark three-piece suit. She, however, had a lovely, gentle smile. Slightly overweight, with big hands and a round face, she reminded me of my grandfather. Looking at her kind eyes, I immediately felt a sense of love and connection with her.

However, what really struck me was their surroundings. Behind them was their house: dilapidated with paint peeling off, there could be no question that they were very poor. My great-grandfather was a farm labourer who farmed for others. As is the case today, the pay was meagre. This meant that only one of their sons, my grandfather's eldest brother, was educated. He eventually became a diplomat.

My grandfather only made it through primary school after which he also had to go work on the farm. He would later marry my grandmother who had inherited a small piece of land which enabled him to farm and feed the family.

As a small child, I was never aware that my grandparents were poor. They didn't have running water or electricity until I was already in my late teens, yet there was so much love, laughter and lovely food that I only realised as an adult how little money they had.

As I stared at the photo of my great-grandmother, I started to wonder whether my anxiety about money went further than just my upbringing. Could it be that apart from the lessons learnt from my immediate family, I had inherited a deep trauma from my ancestors? Even though I had so much more, did I still carry within me the fear of generations of women not knowing if they would be able to feed themselves and their children?

I knew that, although some people still dismiss this, scientists increasingly accept that we carry some knowledge or genetic memory inherited from at least 30 previous generations.

The penny finally dropped. I realised that despite all the work I had done through the years, deep in my DNA I was still carrying generations of fears and anxiety about money!

A few days later when I mentioned it to the women in the Women's Circle, many nodded in agreement and shared their own family histories of poverty. From their own struggles with money, it was clear that many women carry this deep inter-generational wound.

Back at my desk I took a deep breath. I knew it was time to break that trauma cycle once and for all. I knew that it meant accepting that I carried this ancient wound inside me and that it would most probably never disappear. This awareness would help me to recognise and name the fear when it reared its very unpleasant head.

I knew that I also had to be brave, without being reckless, I had to work hard at believing that I would always have the resources to make money.

"Mum, you always panic about money, yet you always find a way to make it," my daughter had said on many occasions to me. I knew she was right, but I had to find the inner strength to believe it.

In order to affirm that belief, I knew that I had to begin spending money on what my soul needed. At that moment my soul was asking me to travel. Perhaps not for six months, but at least for two.

I looked back at the sheet of paper. Could I afford it? I realised I could. I would not be able to contribute my annual tax allowance to my retirement fund, but so what? If I had died from ovarian cancer the previous year, what use would the retirement fund have been? Yes, my financial advisor would give me a long lecture about not being able to keep up my lifestyle when I got older, but frankly, I had had enough of all the fear-based talk from guys dealing with retirement investments.

Instead, I thought about the small "travel" petal on my vision board. It had been a bit of an afterthought at the time, but now I knew that the physical journey needed to take centre stage in my emotional and spiritual journey.

I had no choice but to spend the money.

It was time to bury the bag lady once and for all.

Over the next few days, despite burying the bag lady, I still doubted the wisdom of the trip. My daughter announced that she was pregnant and we were all over the moon, but she was struggling health-wise. How could I leave her? I also worried about my clients. Would they not just move to another political analyst? And of course, what about my dogs?

Yet, I kept looking at my vision board with its affirmation of my need for silence and retreat, dealing with the things that were holding me back, deepening my spiritual practice, looking after my body and making time to write. I eventually came to accept that the trip was not only a deeply needed act of self-love, but a necessity for my physical and emotionally healing.

I also knew that the bigger internal journey that I was about to undertake required saying painful goodbyes to some of the men who had played a significant role in my life.

Bennie

I decided to start my journey in South Africa on a luxury train. I had previously done the 1000-mile train journey from Cape Town to Pretoria with my son before he left to take up a position in Ireland. Now, I wanted to do it with my daughter before her baby arrived.

For four glorious days, time slowed down as we watched the landscape sweep past. Between the meals, I had a lot of time for reflection. Once, whilst staring out the window, I suddenly remembered the unpleasant experience of waking up from the anaesthetic after my operation. I relived how I had struggled to be fully present and how my body was shaking from the shock and extreme pain.

Then, I had another flashback from an operation 50 years before. I was about four years old when my tonsils were removed. I vividly recalled the face of the surgeon, his colourful skullcap and the bright theatre lights. Then a deep sadness filled me as I remembered waiting for my dad to come and visit me.

He never came.

My mum and my biological dad, Bennie, married when they were both at university. From what she told me, he was a very handsome man and had lots of ambitious dreams. This was a big attraction for my mum, who was desperate to escape the small farming and mining community she came from.

I was born a few years later, but by then the wheels had started to come off for my dad. He drank too much and abused prescription drugs, which were readily available to him as a pharmacist. Eventually, my mum took the brave step and divorced him.

Afterwards he would dip in and out of my life. As determined by the divorce agreement I started to visit him from the age of five during school holidays. I would take the two-hour flight on my own and then spend between three and five weeks with him and his second wife, Dawn. These holidays were filled with chaos and at times terror, as my dad struggled to cope with the emotional stress of having me there. Dawn was lovely and tried her best to shield me from it all, but the holidays left deep scars on me.

At the age of thirteen, after a particularly chaotic holiday, I decided to no longer visit him. Legally, I finally had a say. I never saw my dad again until a brief meeting four years later when I needed his signature for a passport.

About a year after that visit to Kimberley, where he lived, he phoned me at my university residence. He had been calling from time to time – usually when he was in an emotional, drunken stupor. It was before the time of cell phones, so to my embarrassment, the public phone was always answered by fellow students in the residence, who had to deal with his initial abuse and obscenities.

On that particular night he was calm and eerily friendly. After inquiring how I was, he asked me to sign over a life insurance policy he was obliged by the divorce agreement to maintain for me. Since he was short of money, he wanted a payout. Slightly in jest I responded: "Ok, if you will sign me off." There was a short silence and then he said: "Ok."

Just like that.

"Ok."

A few days later he flew down and we went to the local magistrate's court. I did not want my mum there so went on my own. My dad was already at the courthouse. Once in front of the magistrate, I asked him to tell my dad to never get in touch with me again. The magistrate looked sharply at my dad and said: "I'm not sure what is going on here, but I know it is not good. So, do the right thing now."

After the proceedings were over, we walked out of the magistrate's court together. There was a long path with rose bushes on either side. When we got to the end of the path, I had to turn left to get to my car, and he turned right.

"Bye…" I whispered.

He said nothing.

After a few steps I looked back, desperately hoping that he would turn around at least one last time.

He didn't.

That was the last time I saw my dad.

That night, clearly upset and drunk, he called me. He

lashed out at me. "You think you are so great, but let me assure you, I know that you will never be a success. Never. You will fail in life and will never achieve anything."

I tried to argue back, but there was nothing I could say that would stop his torrent of abuse.

That was the last time we spoke.

In 1992 I received a call from his wife to tell me he had died. I shed no tears and didn't go to his funeral. I had closed that door. The only way I could figure out how to survive emotionally was not to have any contact with him or his family. At times, my mum would encourage me to try and make contact with his sister, my aunt, who lived close by, but the mere thought of opening that door again created enormous fear in me.

Then in the months after my operation things changed. Increasingly, I started to think about him. One night my mum sat down with me and tried to give me a more positive version of my biological dad. This succeeded only partially because most of the narrative again revolved around the hurt and chaos he caused.

Yet, I started to think and wonder about him more and more. I wasn't sure why. Was it the fact that I had to deal with my own mortality in such an intense way when they discovered the growth, or was it because of a grandchild in the making that had created a need to reconnect with my biological lineage?

Fearfully, I decided to reach out to one of my cousins, who

had found me via LinkedIn a few years previously. At the time I accepted the connection request but didn't communicate any further.

Before I spoke to her, I made a list of what I was hoping for: I wanted to see if anyone had some photos of my dad, since I only had three photos of him, dating back to when I was small. I wanted to know where he was buried, so I could visit his grave. I also wanted to get the contact details of his wife. Lastly, I wanted to try and complete the family tree, so I needed information on my grandparents.

For emotional safety, I decided to WhatsApp her rather than phone.

She responded immediately. Over the next two weeks we would discuss our shared childhood memories. Some were happy ones of days on my grandparents' farm. Others were darker. We skirted around them with only cursory references to the mental health issues and addiction that plagued not only my dad, but other family members.

One night, my cousin sent me some pictures of my grandparents. I zoomed in – trying to remember. My grandfather was familiar to me, my grandmother not so much. Yet, I was struck by how fashionable she looked – even in old age. It made me smile.

However, there were no photos of my dad. My cousin had asked her dad and brother, but neither had any. She then told me that Dawn had passed away two years earlier. She gave me the contact details of her only surviving relative –

a nephew – but when I tried to call him, the number had been discontinued. I also found out that my dad had been cremated and no-one could tell me what had happened to his ashes.

Late one night, I googled his name. Nothing. It was as if he had never existed.

I then tried to get dates and names to try and compile a family tree. Eventually I managed to get the full names of my grandparents as well as my grandmother's date of birth, but nothing more.

During this time, I texted my mum asking for my dad's year of birth. "1940," she responded. I stared at the text as a realisation hit me: my dad had died in 1992, meaning that he was only 52 years old – just a few years younger than me when he died. A sadness went through me. What an incredible waste of a life.

This whole process of discovery unsettled me. Dark dreams disrupted my sleep as old wounds were opened. I also felt that I was making no progress and that despite the grief this was causing me, I would not get any answers to my questions.

A few weeks after my initial contact with my cousin, my mum gave me a graduation photo of my dad. I had briefly seen it years before, but now I studied it closely in the hope of finding something familiar in him. Then I saw it. His nose. Like mine it was slightly smaller on the left side. A flood of love and sadness went through my body and I became tearful.

I did after all belong somewhere. I did carry something of him. Something visible. He did really exist.

That night I showed the photo to my daughter. "Wow! You look a lot like him," she responded.

I always knew that I didn't look like my mother. I don't think I look a lot like my dad – but at least now, after three decades of deliberately cutting myself off from my paternal lineage, I felt some connection with him.

There was also some success with the family tree. I have inherited a genetic condition called Porphyria from my dad. It has had very little impact on my life, apart from having to be very careful with medication (many of which are contra-indicated and can result in a severe and very dangerous reaction).

In the 1960's a geneticist from Dublin, Dr Jeffrey Dean, discovered that this particular strain of porphyria was brought to South Africa in 1688 by an orphan from Rotterdam, called Adriaantjie Jacobs.

Apparently, the Dutch East India company had some difficulty with their all-male employees in South Africa, who became a bit too familiar with the local women, so they decided to send a group of women from Holland as brides for the men. Adriaantjie was only 15 years old when she married one of them.

Dr Dean had done phenomenal work on tracing porphyria's family tree, but I had no idea if my lineage would link up with that tree. With the little information I had of my grandparents, I contacted a family friend who did genealogical research. A few weeks later, he sent me an email and there it was... a straight line through nine generations leading back to Adriaantjie.

I studied the family tree for hours. I wondered about some of my female ancestors who had died young, leaving babies behind. I felt sad for one who had lost his dad at the age of two and wondered if his mum's new husband was kind to them.

I would never know the answers of course, but somehow, seeing their names, dates of birth and death, as well as where they had lived, gave me some comfort. I belonged... not only to this lineage, but also to this country that I loved so dearly, going back almost 400 years.

On day two of our train journey, we got off for an excursion in Kimberley, the town where my dad was living the last time I had visited him to get my passport application signed. Although I had found out from my cousin that he had moved to Johannesburg later, to me it was the last place I associated him with.

Kimberley is known for the deepest (240 meter) hole excavated by hand in the world. Between 1871 and 1914 about 50,000 men dug a 17 hectare-wide hole in search of diamonds, many of them paying with their lives. Today there is a lookout point and museum, which we visited.

At the hole, I waited until I was alone. Then I took out a little red ribbon I had brought with me and tied it to the balustrades.

"Dad," I whispered. "I have come here to tell you that I was a success after all. I have achieved a lot professionally and I have raised two amazing children. So, your curse of that last night did not work. However, I want to be free of the pain and doubt that you caused me. I no longer want to feel that I have to prove you wrong. So, by leaving this ribbon here, I am cutting the dark and hurtful ties between us today."

I felt a bit dizzy as I looked at the ribbon fluttering in the wind.

I then added: "Thank you for giving me life. I love you."

I stood for a few more minutes in the blazing sunlight and listened to the beautiful calls of two fish eagles echoing against the deep cliffs below me.

Then I turned around.

I was done.

Weeks later, I was walking around a lake in Wales. Out of the blue, I thought about my dad. I thought about all the dreams he'd had. For the previous few days, I had been thinking and writing about daring to dream my own dreams. I realized that I have inherited good qualities from both of my parents. From my mum I got the determination and courage to be fully in this world and the drive to make things happen. But, my need to dream, to create and be part of change...that I got from my dad.

Philip

On the morning of day four the train halted for breakfast at a little town called Klerksdorp. "Let's toast Grandpa Philip," said my daughter, as she lifted her glass of orange juice into the air.

Philip wasn't always my dad, but he became my dad.

I have a vague memory of the first time he came to me and my mum's flat and took her out for dinner. On my three-and-a-half-year-old memory that made a big impact.

When they got married a few months later, I was not in a good mood. I didn't object to the marriage; in fact, I was excited. However, my mum had dressed me in a (very fashionable at the time) knitted pant suit. I wanted to wear a dress. When my original plans to boycott the wedding didn't work, I resorted to glaring at the camera in all the wedding photographs.

A year later, Philip brought me to the gardens of the Moedersbond Hospital in Pretoria. Children were not allowed to visit inside but he pointed at the window where my mum was standing with my new little sister.

Shortly after, my mum asked if I would mind calling Philip "dad". I didn't, and so – effortlessly, we became a family.

Whilst my biological dad sucked at fatherhood, Philip provided the quiet, constant security and safety that all kids need.

Philip was a genius. He had a phenomenal intellect. He was sixteen years old when he went to university and a few years later got a doctorate in nuclear physics. He speed-read a few books a day. Dinners and lunches at our house were always filled with deeply – sometimes heated – intellectual conversations. Lazy thinking was not an option, a huge gift to any child.

As a lecturer in Applied Mathematics at the University of Stellenbosch, he was deeply committed to his students. Teaching was important to him – with his children too. He spent hours reading books and teaching chess to my sisters and when we asked him a question, he would get the relevant book and give us a passage to read. If we thought that we could take a mathematical short cut by asking him to do a calculation for us, he would insist that we did it ourselves and to report back how we had got to the answer.

During the last few years of his life, he mentored young students to help get their academic articles published.

But he was also willing to learn.

On the day of the 1994 election, I went home for a quick dinner between political responsibilities. We got involved in a heated discussion and I, with all the arrogance of my youth, challenged him to step out of the comfort of his intellectualism and to "get involved and do something."

A few months later, some of the ANC people in his area told me how impressed they were with my dad. Unbeknown to me, he had joined the local Reconstruction and

Development Programme forum and was playing a huge role there. That led to his involvement with various NGO's – to the point that the endless phone calls from people who were looking for "comrade" Philip drove my mum crazy.

His deep interest in current affairs continued right to the end. A few days before his death, he called me and raised his deep concern about the effect of the COVID-19 epidemic on the country and especially the economy.

Despite Philip's intellectualism, there was also a deeply emotional, soft side to him. One of my lasting memories from childhood is of him sitting on our beds and gently stroking our backs until we fell asleep.

On the morning of his death, in June 2020, he stroked my mum's back just before he got up to juice some oranges for her.

These loving deeds for his wife of 49 years were the last things he did before his phenomenal brain started bleeding.

Philip du Toit Fourie was my dad... my *real* dad.

In a world that was collectively struggling for breath, we battled to organize a memorial for him during the COVID restrictions of level 5 lockdown. In the end we had a beautiful morning with just his closest friends on the slopes of the Stellenbosch mountains that he loved so much. Circumstances forced simplicity and humbleness – exactly what he would have wanted, because my dad was humble – so humble that he had always insisted that he made very little – if any – contribution to the world.

And yet through the stories that others told us after his death it became clear that – without knowing it – he had had a deep impact on many.

The most moving example came from an email a few weeks after his death, from someone I had never met:

"I'm sorry about the loss of your dad," it read. *"I also had to bury my dad and no one knows how you feel. Your dad was my lecturer in Applied Mathematics in 1993 at the University of Stellenbosch and he was in his (subtle) way the best lecturer I ever had. He once wrote all the names of Elizabeth Taylor's husbands on the blackboard and we asked what it was about. In his dry manner he answered that this was the Hollywood version of the Taylor Series and so made a very difficult bit of mathematics easy for us.*

One day, I saw him cycling past the university residence I lived in. He stopped, got off his bicycle and picked up paper in Piet Retief Street and threw it in a rubbish bin. I still remember it to this day – and I always pick up rubbish. When I work on construction sites, I pick up rubbish and when people give me puzzled looks, I just smile and think: 'I had a great teacher.' Your dad has left a lasting impression on me."

As he did on me.

On the day of his memorial I said:

"Thank you, Dad, for taking me on – I know it could not have been easy. Thank you for making my life stable and safe. Thank you for walking me down the aisle when I got married and being there for all the important days in my life. Thank you for being (furiously) on my side when I got divorced. Thank you for being such a proud and loving grandfather to my children. And thank you for being such a good husband to my mum – for making her happy again and giving her faith in life after her first marriage.

I will miss you terribly."

Almost two years on I still missed him terribly, but unlike that of my biological dad, it is a "clean" and uncomplicated grief. Looking out the train window at the town where he was born, I thought how different it was from the ocean and mountains which surrounded him during the last few decades of his life.

I raised my glass and tapped it gently against my daughter's – and whispered silently: "I still miss you so much dad. How I wish I could have told you about this journey I am on!"

Gerry

I decided to begin the overseas leg of my journey in Ireland. I was apprehensive about it. I had visited Ireland numerous times since I left in 2013 and every time it had brought back a flood of trauma and pain. As someone said to me once: "Ireland is soaked with your tears."

On 30 April 1990 I had found Gerry on the floor of our bedroom. The man that I loved so deeply was cold and unresponsive. He had died a few hours earlier from a heart attack.

In that moment, I could feel the world starting to spin faster and faster – out of control. I knew instinctively that the world as I had known it would never be the same. What I thankfully did not yet know was that it would also be true of my inner world.

The first night I spent with Gerry, I got out of bed and sat in the dark for a long time. I was worried. On the surface we were very different – in fact if I had met him a few years before, I would not have considered a relationship with him.

Yet, I had a strong sense that my journey to Ireland, my divorce – perhaps my whole life, had led me to him. Staring out at the trees in Herbert Park below his apartment and listening to the chiming of the church bells nearby, I knew I had a decision to make. I could follow my head, get dressed and leave. Or, I could take an enormous leap of faith, trust my heart and get back into bed.

I stayed.

For two glorious years, Gerry and I shared the most extraordinary love. He saw and loved me for who I was, and I felt the same about him. I relaxed physically and emotionally into the warm embrace of our love. Two nights before he died, I wrote in my diary: "I am so happy. Things are finally coming together in my life."

Then he died…

I have never known grief that deep. I also did not know how tiring and physical grief was. Added to the immensity of the pain of his loss was the fact that it all played out in public. From about 30 minutes after I phoned the emergency services, to the time I left Ireland three years later, the press remained a constant companion in my life.

Since he was separated, but not yet formally divorced, I had to fight to be part of the rituals of saying goodbye – rituals that are so important in the healing of grief.

My dreams for the future died with Gerry. For almost a decade I went into survival mode. I had to provide for my children and after returning to South Africa, I focused on re-inventing myself professionally in order to make ends meet.

My political analysis business became very successful, for which I was thankful. Yet, I dared not dream any longer. For me, following my heart posed risks – deadly risks and I was no longer willing to go there.

Perhaps it is no wonder that I was diagnosed a few years later with a left branch bundle block (LBBB) – a benign condition of the heart where the heart doesn't fire correctly.

Of course, over the years, my "handbag of grief" had become lighter. Yet, the pain and grief still denied me the freedom to dream – to imagine a world where I could trust and give in to the longings of my heart.

This was primarily due to the tremendous loss I felt, no longer having Gerry with me. Still, I realized over time that a part of me did not want to let go of the pain, since I was fearful that I would forget him and the love we shared. That would be a betrayal that I could not live with.

In the months after the hysterectomy, I dreamt repeatedly about Gerry. Every time I would wake up in tears. I knew that it was my mind and possibly my body too, urging me to deal with the grief that I felt so deeply, but I didn't know how to do that.

One morning after yet another fretful and tearful night, I thought – really thought – about Gerry. I tried to remember his body – every single line and freckle. The fact that I was able to recall it all in such detail brought an enormous sense of relief. If I was able to remember after more than ten years, perhaps it was safe to let go. As much as it scared me, I knew I had to go to Ireland to say goodbye.

I first stayed with my friend Brid. The first few nights after Gerry's death she had slept next to me in the sitting room and held my hand when I couldn't face the bed he and I had shared. She would also later bravely accompany me to his funeral and the inquest into his death, and she'd spend the day with me every year on the anniversary of his death.

After a few days in Dublin, we decided to go away for a night around St Patrick's Day. We travelled to West Meath, which is regarded as the ancient centre of Ireland, where the high kings and queens ruled. In a light drizzle we stopped at a well that was dedicated to St Brigid.

After a short ritual, I sat down next to the well and, like pilgrims through the centuries, I dipped my hands into the icy water. Then I prayed that my writing would be blessed. I also prayed to be released from those ties to Gerry that were holding me back from the fulness of life.

Later that night, when we came back from dinner, the full moon rose majestically over the freezing fields of Ireland.

"You know that the full moon is about letting go, right?" said Brid.

On our way back to Dublin the next day, Brid asked if I wanted to visit Gerry's grave. I wasn't sure. The grave was a particularly painful reminder of the past for me. On the day of his funeral, I had stood back as his wife, children, family and friends said goodbye. The inscription on the gravestone came from his estranged wife, not me. Even though I had gone there many times, I had never felt any real connection to Gerry there. In fact, the mere idea that his body was somewhere under the icy ground freaked me out.

Yet, I knew I had to say goodbye. Not to him or our love, but to the pain I now wanted to be free from. I walked slowly to the familiar grave site right at the entrance of the cemetery and sat down on the side of Gerry's gravestone. Wary of curious looks from passersby, I dropped my long hair around my face and whispered "Hi!" I immediately felt my eyes well up.

With my tears flowing freely, I told Gerry that I needed to be free, that I would forever love him and hoped that we would reconnect one day in another form. Still, for now I had to live in this world and couldn't do that if I was still so sad about losing him. I asked to be released from all that was holding me back. Then I got up and walked back to the car where Brid was waiting. With every step I took, I felt a bit lighter.

Two days later Brid and I visited Herbert Park. Gerry and I had spent many happy hours there in the year before he died. In the winter we would sit around the pond in the soft sunlight watching the ducks and sea gulls. Days before he died, we picnicked under the cherry trees and marvelled at the spectacular show of blossoms.

After his death I had a bench erected there in his honour. The little plaque with a quote from a song from the movie Moulin Rouge reads: For Gerry (5/6/1956-30/4/2020). "Season may change winter to spring, but I will love you till the end of time." Melanie

For the months before I moved back to South Africa, it was the place I came to remember Gerry. It was there at the water, amongst the ducks and birds and surrounded by cherry blossoms, that I felt connected to him.

Later, on my visits back to Ireland I would always go back to the bench. More often than not people (usually a group of elderly men) would be sitting on the bench. Even though I knew that Gerry would have loved the old men chewing the cud on "his" bench, I was always a bit sad that I couldn't sit on it myself.

However, on this day – even though all the other benches were occupied – Gerry's bench was empty. For about two hours Brid and I sat in glorious sunshine and reminisced about the past. People walked past and nodded, dogs came to say hello and the ducks paddled around happily.

As we got ready to leave, I looked over to a row of trees in full bloom and thought how much they served as a reminder of the continuing – albeit short lived – beauty of life.

I felt light and free.

A month later, on the day I returned to South Africa, I received a text from Brid. It was late in the evening, but she wanted to say that she'd been thinking of me because of what day it was. For a moment I couldn't understand what she was talking about.

Then it hit me. It was the anniversary of Gerry's death. In between all the chaos of landing back in the country and unpacking, I had forgotten. I waited for the guilt and pain to hit me. It didn't. I suddenly saw Gerry's face and his broad smile in front of me.

I sighed a big sigh of relief.

I knew that I would forever love Gerry, that I would never forget the feeling of his embrace or the sound of his heart. I would never stop missing him, but I also wanted to make space for dreams in my heart again – as scary as that might be.

Letting my soul breathe – or not

"Fuck all this 'no mud, no lotus' stuff," I whispered under my breath. "This is too hard!"

As I entered the new year, I wanted to deal with the anxiety-riddled exhaustion that had become my constant companion since the operation. "I'm going to kick the shit out of this, because it is holding me back," I wrote in my diary.

My physical healing was going well, and I had committed to focus more on myself. However, I realised that in order to walk the road of healing with integrity and to fully respond to the calling of my soul, I needed to carve out time for spiritual reflection. I had to create space and time (and find the discipline) to sit in silence – something which is always difficult in our noisy world.

Early in January just a few days before my decision to travel, it was announced that the Vietnamese Buddhist monk Thich Nhat Hanh had died. Even though he was 95 years old and had been sick for a while, I was filled with sadness. It was just a few days after Archbishop Tutu's death, and it felt to me as if all the good people were dying.

I had once attended an event with Thay, as he was affectionately known, in Dublin in 2012. It was an extraordinary evening. The hall was packed to the rafters which, given the fact that around 80% of Irish people regard themselves as Catholic, surprised me.

Thich Nhat Hanh was surrounded by other monks and nuns from his order, and together they led a deep meditation. I have been to many religious meetings in my life, but I had never experienced anything like it. The silence of hundreds of people meditating was deafening.

The energy that Thich Nhat Hanh generated through gentle speech, chanting and the beating of a prayer drum was electrifying. As people left they walked silently and slowly. I was blown away.

Thich Nhat Hanh is known for bringing the practice of mindfulness to the West. I knew roughly what mindfulness was. I had read many of his books. With a focus on breathing, the aim was to stay in the moment.

Even though I have tried to meditate for most of my adult life, I found mindfulness almost impossible. My brain was just too busy. In fact, I kinda liked that my mind was able to store so many things at the same time and that I could multi-task.

I never made the connection to the exhaustion that was a perpetual presence in my life. Of course, my demanding professional life, combined with raising two children, played a huge role, but there was also a mental exhaustion that often led to anxiety.

As I watched the live stream on the internet of the monks and nuns in Korea and Plum Village in France paying their last respects to Thich Nhat Hanh, I felt a strong pull to visit them. For years I had been looking at photos of Thich Nhat Hanh at Plum Village, the monastery he established near

Bordeaux in France. I had always felt drawn to it, but I wasn't sure that I was ready for it. Now I decided to see if they would allow people to stay for a while.

A friendly nun emailed back that they would receive a small group of people at the end of April. I took it as a sign and paid the donation for the two weeks.

After spending a week with my son in France and Spain, I took the train to Bordeaux and from there to St Foy le Grande to get to Plum Village. It was a local train which stopped at numerous stations, and at one of them a red-headed woman boarded. I gestured to her that I had space across from me and she plonked herself down, looked at my luggage and exclaimed: "It looks like you are also going to Plum Village!"

I laughingly confirmed that I was. She introduced herself as Felicity and exclaimed: "Wouldn't it be fun if we were in the same room?" Amazingly, that is exactly what happened. Felicity, who is a bubbly person with the most beautiful soul, was a godsend, since the time at Lower Hamlet (the female side of Plum Village) turned out to be very challenging.

Within a day, I knew that it was not a comfortable space for me. I wasn't sure what the problem was. I love silence, so the 14 hours of "noble silence" per day was not a problem at all. On my last trip to Bali, for example, I had benefitted greatly from a lengthy silent retreat.

When I announced to family and friends that I was going to do a five-day silent retreat they were sceptical. "You are definitely going to be kicked out," said a family member, a sentiment shared by the rest of the doubting Thomases. Okay, it is perhaps understandable given that I do – and always have – made a living out of talking, but it could be exactly because of my noisy occupation that a few days at The Bali Silent Retreat Centre appealed so much to me.

The simple centre is based in rural northwest Bali, close to the mountains. The scenery is breathtaking, with rustic wooden huts surrounded by rice fields. Although guided meditation and yoga were available, there was no obligation to do anything. There were very few rules: no phones – there was in any case no reception or Wi-Fi – no smoking, no food in the huts (because food attracted mice which in turn attracted snakes) and of course, no talking.

Contrary to my family and friends' predictions, I had no problem being on my own in silence. However, being amongst people (at mealtimes for example) and not saying a word was rather difficult at first. It was challenging to be with people for five days without having a clue what their names were, where they were from or what they did for a living. It became a little personal game to try and guess their nationality and whether they were friendly – based on whether they made eye contact and smiled.

There were a few other challenges. The huts were open at the top and despite having a mosquito net, the mozzies and I held an epic re-enactment of the Battle of Blood River every evening – which they won. Despite my love for the African bush, the Indonesian sounds at night were deafening and kept me awake for a long time. Initially the darkness made me feel a bit unsafe – an occupational hazard of being South African, I guess.

Then there was the episode with the caramelized snakeskin. Every day, delicious vegetarian food was served buffet style. Next to the table there was always a blackboard identifying the different dishes by number. The second morning at breakfast, I scanned the board: 1) Spinach frittata, 2) Kitchree, 3) Caramelized snakeskin... "WHAT?" My brain froze.

I swirled around to have a look at the table. There was the egg thing at no 1, the kitchree at no 2, and something white and leathery floating in a brown syrup at no 3. It didn't look like snakeskin to me, but then again, I have never eaten snakeskin – caramelized or otherwise.

My brain – which had finally started to slow down – went into overdrive. "I thought this was a vegetarian place, how can they kill snakes? Did one of them accidently follow a mouse into a hut and that was the end of him or her? No... that can't be right either. Maybe I should ask someone? Shit! I can't, I'm not allowed to speak!"

After a few minutes of frantic mental activity, I decided to just give no 3 a skip and not even look at it again. I turned back to the board to read the rest of the items, in the hope that they would be less exotic.

The next line read "...fruit."

I paused. My eyes went up to no 3 again.

"Caramelized snakeskin ...fruit!"

Turns out someone with an odd sense of humour had written "fruit" in very small writing with a smiley face next to it on the next line. Phew!

Dietary mishap aside, the Bali retreat was one of the most amazing five days of my life. Within an hour, I was walking more slowly and treading more softly in order not to make a noise. By the second day my brain had started to calm down and by day four I started to have brief moments of non-thinking.

I ate much more slowly and not only tasted the food properly but consumed significantly less. Because I had slowed down, I started to notice little flowers and little insects. I heard the birds singing and the beetles buzzing. I even stopped panicking when I didn't have my phone in my hand.

This lasted for a while, but of course after my return, when I was back into my noisy world of phone calls, TV, newspapers, and people, it gradually evaporated.

Hoping that I could find some of that peace again was why I had decided to go to Plum Village. Yet, being there, I felt anything but peaceful. In fact, I felt deeply unsettled.

The rigid routine and long hours of meditation reminded me of my deep resentment and aversion to organised religion.

I had studied theology at Stellenbosch University, and

after that I knew that I would never become a minister in the Dutch Reformed Church. Not only did they disapprove of the ordination of women – something that has since changed – but I disapproved of their politics.

For decades the Dutch Reformed Church had provided the theological justification and underpinning for the evil policy of Apartheid. Like most white children – and adults for that matter – I never questioned the church. It was only in my second year at university, having been being exposed to political exiles in the United Kingdom, that I understood the extent of the church's collusion with the Apartheid state. I felt deeply betrayed by those who I had put on a pedestal for so long.

I also realised how dangerous organised religion could be. I knew it wasn't true of all communities of faith, but even a cursory look across the world confirmed that religious zealots played (and continue to play) a huge role in many destructive and violent conflicts.

So, I abandoned organised religion and my dream of becoming a minister. I knew I had to find another path.

Over the years I continued to search for an authentic spiritual life and amongst others, tried to deepen my understanding and practice of meditation.

I liked much of what I read about Buddhism – especially its commitment to do no harm or cause suffering to humans, animals or nature. This was one of the things I found attractive at the monastery.
However, even though Buddhists insist that their practice

is not a religion, but a way of life, the long hours of collective meditation, the bowing to the statue of the Buddha and the strict rules at the monastery all brought up uncomfortable memories.

In addition, I was reminded of my deep hatred of being told what to do. Even as a child I had always rebelled when given instructions. So when I was told to clean the monastery for up to four hours per day as part of "service meditation" I felt angry resistance rise in me. It's not that I have a problem with cleaning, nor that I was being told to do hard labour after paying more than a thousand Euro to be there. It was the fact that I was instructed to do something. "Ask me nicely and I'm all yours," I thought angrily. "Instruct me – and I'm out of here."

After a few days, I walked into a nearby vineyard and called my daughter.

"Why don't you just leave?" she asked.

I felt the panic rise in me.

"How can I?" I asked.

"Why not? You paid for it. It's not your thing. Just leave."

After the call, I contemplated leaving. Others who also found it too difficult were departing on a daily basis, so should I? I knew I wouldn't. I couldn't.

"What would the nuns and other women think of me?" I kept thinking.

So I struggled on.

It was only towards the end of the time there that I realised that my "monastic experience" was, after all, teaching me a needed lesson, albeit the opposite of what I had expected:

It was insisting that I deal with my *goodgirlness*.

Deadly politeness

"How is it possible that I didn't feel anything?" I asked the surgeon.

I had read the pathologist's report, which included a picture of the tumour next to a ruler – presumably to rule out any exaggeration on his part.

I have never been good with measurements and distances, which is why my car's satellite navigation system drives me crazy. "Turn right in 200 meters," the woman with the British accent would say, presumably trying to be helpful. "How far is 200 meters?" I would reply, feeling slightly panicked. She would then (rudely) fall silent as I start to sweat in anticipation of her urgent and (I'm convinced) irritated: "Turn right now, turn right NOW!" and then the exasperated: "make a U-turn and head south-east."

"WHERE THE FUCK IS SOUTH-EAST???"

How I wished they still made maps.

I knew that there would also not be a map for the emotional journey I was about to embark on, but if there was any hope of finding my emotional direction again, I needed to find answers. I had always been conscientious about my health; I had done all the recommended regular check-ups and I have always been very aware of my body. Did I miss something? Did I do something wrong? Was there something more I should have done?

I needed a reference point so that I could visualise the thing that had caused so much mayhem in my life.

I had earlier measured the long side of my credit card. That was just over 8 cm – about the same size as the growth. The flatness confused me – I needed something round for comparison. I then googled the size of a cricket ball which turned out to be just under 8 cm. My son used to play cricket, so balls frequently came flying through the windows of our house. I could get my head around a cricket ball.

"How could something the size of a cricket ball grow inside me without any warning signals?" I asked again.

"Actually, it was bigger than a cricket ball – more like a small grapefruit," replied the surgeon.

I thought about it for a minute. I imagined a grapefruit growing on the tree-like structure of my ovary. I liked that a lot more than a hard, red cricket ball.

Fruit and sports equipment aside, why was I not in any pain beforehand?

"Well, your organs accommodated the growth," explained the surgeon. "They politely created space in the belief that it might be a pregnancy."

So there it was.

I have polite organs. So polite in fact that they could have killed me.

"This," explains the surgeon, "is why so many gynaecological cancers (ovarian, uterine and cervical) are only detected at an advanced stage. They are sneaky and grow silently with the cooperation of the adjacent organs."

"Now isn't that just grand?" I thought ironically. "Even my organs had become good girls".

Like most women, I learnt early in life the rules of being a good girl. Don't be too loud, eat nicely, never sit with your legs open, be helpful, be friendly. Anger isn't nice and nobody likes a know-it-all (except if you are a man, of course).

Being competitive, I wasn't going to be just the good girl that was expected of me, I was going to be the best. Forget superwoman I was going to be supergoodgirl!

Of course, below all of the goodgirlness is the need to be liked. I knew intuitively that the road to being liked is to behave, dress and speak a certain way.

Of course, who doesn't like to be liked? Archbishop Tutu once told me that this was his biggest weakness. However, male likeability is linked to performance and achievement. Generally, we like strong, successful men. For women it is different. Girls learn very young that in order to be liked they need to be a "good" and the definition of "good" for girls is very different from that for boys.

Details might differ between different societies and religions, but in general they are based on the belief that women are weaker than men and thus need to be protected. Many religions and cultures also see women as temptresses or seducers of men. Even worse, many view women's bodies and their cycles as impure. Unsurprisingly girls internalise these views – helped also by mothers who uncritically enforce these attitudes on their daughters.

Even though I was determined to be as good a girl as I could be, even as a child I knew that there was a high price to pay for goodgirlness. As I grew older, I came to understand that a certain amount of emotional and physical freedom would be sacrificed. Yes, goodgirlness resulted in being liked, but was also a trap which meant that huge parts of my inner life would remain "unused" (to quote Sue Monk Kidd).

A psychologist friend of mine once remarked on how important freedom was to me. I had assumed that it is was equally true for all people. After all, wasn't that what the fight against Apartheid, the civil rights movement and so many wars all over the world were all about?

He agreed, but still insisted that my need for freedom played a key role in my psyche – more so than for many other people.

On reflection, I had to admit that he was right.

Like all people I have a basic need for belonging and connecting, yet freedom is what I crave most. In *Eat, Pray, Love*, Elizabeth Gilbert remarks that every place or person has a word.

My word is freedom.

Even as a young woman I loved the poem, "Warning" by Jenny Joseph. In it she talks about wearing purple and red together once she gets older. She is also determined to do things like sitting on the pavement, learning to spit and picking flowers in other people's gardens.

Something deep inside me resonated with Jenny's words. Not only were purple and red my two favourite colours, but I loved her defiance.

Having said that, I always felt a bit disappointed, since she also talks about having to wait until she is old, although she does acknowledge that it is perhaps good to start practicing a bit so that it doesn't come as too much of a shock for people once she is elderly.

Even though I worked hard at being supergoodgirl, I had always practiced a little – even when it came to sitting on pavements. Literally. One of my favourite activities has always been to sit on the floor in bookshops and page through a pile of books or to lean against a tree in a park and read.

Even when I was an Ambassador, I did exactly that. At lunchtimes on the rare sunny days, I would go to St Stephen's Green Park in the centre of Dublin, kick off my high heels and sit on the grass and the world would disappear while I read for a while. On one occasion I was told that someone had seen me and laid an official complaint. Apparently, I was in breach of diplomatic protocol and insulting the high office that I held.

I ignored the complaint.

I also had no problem defying societal beliefs or authority figures when I truly believed that they were wrong.

I grew up during the height of Apartheid in South Africa. I went to an all-white school, prayed in an all-white church, and lived in an all-white neighbourhood. Despite the fact that whites made up less than 10% of the population, my only contact with people of other races was through our cleaner and gardener.

Even though we were taught at school, university and church that the apartheid system was divinely inspired and sanctioned, I always had a suspicion that this was all a big lie. Even at the age of six, I had a huge argument with my grandparents about the living conditions of workers on their farm.

At school I once pulled a face of disbelief when the headmistress gave a lecture in assembly about "terrorists and savages" burning down the townships a few kilometres away. Afterwards, she asked me why I had pulled a face. I told her that I didn't believe in what she said. She went red in the face poked her finger against my nose and said: "Be careful young, lady!" I just stared her down.

During my first year at university, I finally met South African exiles whilst visiting Wilhelm, who was studying at Oxford University. Listening to their stories changed my world completely and when I returned to South Africa, I was determined to find out more. So, my political journey began.

In 1990, I finally had the opportunity to meet Nelson Mandela. Shortly after his release from prison he paid a visit to Stellenbosch to meet with white academics. For some reason Wilhelm and I were invited too.

At some stage someone introduced us to Mandela. He immediately realised that Wilhelm was the grandson of the man who was responsible for the banning of the ANC and for his own incarceration. Wilhelm wanted to apologise for his family's role, but Mandela, stopped him.

"You only have to realise that your surname will be recognised, and people will listen to what you have to say. You now have to decide if you want to use that for the bigger good," he said.

Then he asked after Wilhelm's grandmother – the widow of the former prime minister. We explained that she had moved to a white homeland that some of the family had created in a remote area of the country.

Mandela nodded and then said: "Please send her my regards. Tell her from one grey head to another that I'm glad she has reached such a good age and that I wish her well."

I was blown away by the grace and forgiving spirit of this great man, who we whites had been taught was the personification of evil. I had been debating for months whether to join the ANC. Now my mind was made up and a few days later, I quietly did so.

A year later when it became known that I – and eventually Wilhelm – were ANC members, all hell broke loose. The press hounded us and the white population hated us. We received endless death threats, people spat on me in the streets or swore at me in shops. We lost all our "friends". Even though this was extremely stressful, I didn't for one second doubt that we had done the right thing.
This was the total antithesis of what it meant to be a good girl at the time, but I couldn't care less. In the face of injustice, I had always been fearless and I truly believed that this was the moral thing to do.

This same spirit lives in me today. I write a weekly column for a big media outlet and never does a week go by without some hate mail. It is always unpleasant, but I never consider giving up.

Speaking out and claiming pavement-sitting freedoms were things I always did, yet even so, I never felt completely free. There was still a quiet yearning deep in my soul for something more.

After my operation, the need to give attention to this longing became more and more urgent. It felt like a constant heartbeat in my ears – "be free, be free." This came to a crescendo at that monastery in France when the physical rules and routines caused me to face a deeper emotional crisis.

One day, sitting – or rather hiding – in the forest, I

suddenly realised that the "be free, be free" heartbeat I felt was what Glennon Doyle calls the "this-is-not-it-whisper."

But if this was not it, what was?

I knew that I would only find the answer when I removed the barriers of fear and shame that prevented me from claiming the freedom that I was craving.

I had to shed my old skin, and shake off the scabs of deep-seated fears and self-imposed limitations before I would be able to claim a new me. It would continue to be a painful process of self-discovery through brutal honesty.

It would require the warrior woman in me to pick up my sword and bravely fight old demons, whilst at the same time gently heal painful wounds from the past. This meant venturing into an unknown world, without any clarity or certainty about where I would end up.

It scared me, but I knew it was time. I could no longer delay. I was ready.

I turned 55 while I was at the monastery. It was a deeply introspective day for me. I realised that I had spent over five decades being goodgirl and I was sick of it.

So, I gave myself permission to withdrew from the activities at the monastery and only do what felt healing and soothing to me. Of course, it caused enormous anxiety in the beginning, but gradually the panic became less as I was able to silence goodgirl's voice more and more.

I knew that it would take time – possibly a lifetime of battle with goodgirl to rid me of her insistent critical voice and finger pointing – much like with my school principal so many years ago. Still, I was making a start. After all, she was not the only superhero that I had gone into battle with.

Melanie Verwoerd

Slaying super woman

Despite being a goodgirl, I never ever saw myself as inferior to men. I come from a line of strong women, who never allowed men to dominate them. Yet, patriarchy is so invasive that if it doesn't get you on one front, it will get you on another.

One morning, shortly before I had embarked on my trip, I was reflecting on the many wounds patriarchy inflicted on women. I felt a deep sense of unease inside me. Yet, I knew intuitively that there was something more.

My mother had come to visit the previous day. Like a woman possessed I tidied and cleaned before she arrived. "Why do I always do that?" I wondered. I put myself under so much strain every time my family comes to visit that in the end, I don't even enjoy it. I knew they didn't expect it, yet at 55, I was still driving myself crazy before every visit.

I was aware that goodgirl played a role, especially in my attempts to still please my mother, but that was not the full story.

The Aha! moment came when I realised that I was not only carrying a patriarchal wound, but also "a feminist wound" – an "I-have-to-do-it-all-and-do-it-perfectly" wound.

I have a phenomenal mother. She was one of the first women in South African to get a Master's degree in computer science at a time when computers were still room sized. She kept on working even while running the household and raising three girls.

I really love my mother and am very thankful for all that she gave me. Her life inspired much of my sisters' and my success.

However, as with most women who had experienced the feminist revolution of the late 60's and 70's, my mum just took on more. The burden of the household and children remained largely on her shoulders, but she was determined to have a career, and the message from society was that it had to be done perfectly.

It was as if the subconscious message was: if you want to be a feminist and have a career – fine, but you better not slip up on the home front.

Through the years, I had absorbed that message. I was determined to be successful and follow my dreams, but I felt obligated to also maintain the traditional, domestic roles perfectly.

And so goodgirl grew up to also become superwoman.

I tried to run a perfect house, be the perfect mother, look good and dress well, make my own money (but not too much because that is obscene), be a good Christian (and later, spiritual person), entertainer, cook, baker as well as read books and go to theatre in order to be cultured. Of course, I also aspired to be a brilliant politician and ambassador.

I regularly stretched my physical and mental health to the brink, because I could not face the inevitable shame that would come with "failing" – or what I call the "cupcake phenomenon".

Shortly after the first democratic election in South Africa, parliament was tasked with writing of the new constitution for the country. Writing the constitution was a fantastic experience. There was a real sense of being part of making history. After all, how many people get the chance to help write the founding document of their nation?

As we got closer to the constitutionally binding deadline, tension rose dramatically. There were still many outstanding issues, and the opposition parties were digging in their heels. During the final few weeks, we often worked through the night.

With one day left, I drove back home early one morning to have a quick shower, feed the kids breakfast and take them to pre-school, before heading back to parliament for the final outstanding pieces of work.

As we arrived at the school, the principal, Mrs Prior, met me.

"Melanie, please remember it is your turn for cupcakes tomorrow," she said.

I looked at her in a daze.

"Cupcakes?" Then I remembered. Every Friday, the

children took money to school for charity and bought a cupcake provided by one of the mums.

My head was filled with the constitutional responsibilities of local government, and the whole cupcake business had completely slipped my mind. I explained that I had not slept in days and that we were in the last day of constitutional negotiations. Was there perhaps another mother who could swap with me?

"No!" Mrs Prior insisted.

Apparently, I was the only mother who had not taken a turn, and no, I could also not buy something else like popcorn: it had to be homemade cupcakes. I looked down at my two little ones staring worriedly up at me. Of course, at their age, the constitution meant nothing. Cupcakes, and not being embarrassed, were far more important. So, of course I agreed. How could I not? After yet another long day and night at parliament, I stood at two in the morning in my kitchen icing cupcakes, wondering whether any male MP anywhere in the world had ever done this.

Why did I just not say no?

Because of shame.

Not being able to bake cupcakes like "all the other mothers" would have meant that I failed in my mothering. Could there be any bigger shame than that?

Looking back now, I know that it was ridiculous, but the voices of indoctrination were much more convincing – or perhaps I was just too tired to argue with those voices in myself.

Of course, there were many similar examples of the "cupcake syndrome". My mother-in-law came to our apartment a few weeks after we got married with shopping bags full of food, since she was convinced that I did not feed her beloved son. Instead of telling her that he had two hands and could help himself to food, I felt utterly ashamed and vowed to do better. Believe it or not, I was doing a degree in feminist theology at the time.

I also felt deep shame when my husband once told me how it annoyed him that I would get into comfortable (he called it "sloppy") clothes at home after being dressed up all day for work. Then there was the time the school phoned to ask if we were still picking up our children. I was away on a work trip and my husband had forgotten that it was his turn – yet it was I who felt terrible.

I will also never forget my mother-in-law phoning to tell me that, to her surprise, my children turned out ok. There were many other such examples, and thinking back on them now, I can still feel my cheeks burning with shame.

Strangely, this even applied to my health. I have always worked hard at staying healthy and have read endless books about the topic. I follow a healthy diet and I exercise. Yet, throughout my life, any illness – even the ovarian tumour – felt like a personal failure.

Thinking back over all of this, I felt tears welling up. No wonder I was exhausted. It was too much! Something had to give and together with my marriage it was far too often my health.

Over the next few days, I wondered why a feminist like me would buy into all of this?

When I discussed it with my psychologist friend, he said that Dr Spock's approach to childrearing meant that, "children of the 60's and 70's understood subconsciously that love was transactional. In order for mums to have perfect children – children had to be controlled – thus the need for feeding by the hours and sleep training. So, a false love – where love gets subconsciously associated with being good – is inculcated and in the process the act of self-love gets deeply injured."

I immediately identified with what he said. The constant hum of self-criticism, of "you are not being good enough" together with the voices of superwoman and goodgirl were enough proof that I also carried that psychological wound.

"How do I heal that?" I asked my friend.

"You have to fall in love with yourself. You have to be softer and kinder and shut out the internal critical voice," he responded, "and you have to do what your soul and especially your body ask of you."

I felt my body resisting. Following what my soul wanted was one thing but listening to what my body wanted was a different story. For that I had to trust my body and I certainly did not feel any faith in my body anymore – if I ever had.

Trusting my body

"I feel like my body betrayed me."

Abraham and I were sitting in the cool breeze on my balcony. "I thought we had a deal. I would eat well, exercise, take supplements, not smoke or drink and have regular check-ups. In return my body's only job was to stay healthy – at least with the big stuff." I felt tears welling up. "I feel my body broke the deal. How will I trust her again?"

Abraham looked at me calmly.

"Actually, she didn't," he said. "She kept her side of the bargain. Yes, a growth developed, but it was discovered and against all the odds it wasn't cancer. To me your body really kept the deal."

I wasn't convinced and I kept wondering how to trust my body again. When I found the lump on my knee a while later, my first thought was: "here we go again."

However, I also had to be honest. I really had not had much faith in my body before the operation either.

For more than a decade I had struggled with vertigo (dizziness). It started after I got a very bad blood infection in Kenya at the beginning of 2008. With Kenya in the midst of post-election violence, it was a particularly stressful trip. I was there for UNICEF and as is often the case, I picked up some mysterious infection during my visits to various refugee camps.

Melanie Verwoerd

The sickness worsened rapidly during a few days in Rwanda, where I was hoping to decompress. I eventually went to a doctor, who could only speak French, and since I spoke none, I phoned my GP in Ireland who thankfully had spent a year in Paris. She told me afterwards how concerned she was about my blood results. Despite her warning to stay close to a hospital, I kept working and even climbed up into the mountains to see the famous gorillas.

Back in Ireland, I remained seriously unwell for a long time. Even after I felt better, I had lingering episodes of dizziness, eventually diagnosed as vertigo.

From time to time, I experienced serious bouts of spinning which made it impossible to even sit upright, but mostly the vertigo manifested as a low-level dizziness. To make matters worse, since our bodies don't like to be off-balance, when the vertigo hits you it sends warning or panic signals to the brain. The resulting anxiety has always been the worst part of it for me.

I have tried various forms of therapy and it is much better than it was, but from time to time it still returns. Over the years I have tried to avoid settings that might trigger it. Malls and hairdressers, with all their bright reflections and noise, are uncomfortable. I don't like places with a lot of people, such as shopping queues where I have to stand for a long time. Most annoyingly, vertigo also influences my work. I used to love public speaking, but over the years I started to dread it. Fearful that if I declined invitations, I would never be asked back, I would ask the event organisers for a chair to lean against – pretending that it was part of my "performance". Still, I would be petrified in the run up to an event and when I felt I simply couldn't do it at all, I would think up elaborate excuses.

Increasingly, I no longer felt safe in my body. I even started to see her as a stumbling block or "enemy" who made it difficult for me to do the things I wanted to do.

Nobody knew to what extent I was hampered by this. Yes, my family knew that I would have attacks from time to time, but not even they knew how miserable it made me. The secrecy, of course, only made it worse.

With the arrival of menopause came a whole new string of unpleasant bodily experiences.

As with vertigo, I was determined not to show any weakness – especially not in the male dominated professional world I worked in. I would marvel at the courage of men who would openly discuss their health difficulties and wondered why I couldn't do the same. Of course, feminism and competing in a very masculine world was part of it, but I started to realise that there was more to it – since I didn't even tell my closest female friends.

The answer came in the months after the operation.

Given that the hysterectomy involved open surgery, I needed help for a while afterwards. For the first two days in hospital, I couldn't even get out of bed and needed help from the nursing staff for the smallest thing. I felt like a burden and apologised profusely every time I had to ring for help.

"Mum, you know it's their job?" said my daughter after watching another apologetic ringing of the bell.

By the time I was released from hospital I could, with some effort, go to the bathroom, but had to have someone close by in case I fainted. I was told not to lift anything heavier than 1kg (women are often told – only a cup of tea) for weeks. Bending was impossible – and even opening a sliding door was prohibited.

When I confided in my daughter how much I hated to ask for help, she wanted to know why.

"Because I feel ashamed," I responded without thinking.

She looked at me in disbelief.

"You have had major surgery, why on earth would you feel ashamed?"

I couldn't understand it either, but in the months to come, I would realise that I also felt a deep sense of shame about having vertigo – which was why I hid it so well from others.

Fed up with the way it hampered me, I decided to do whatever it took to deal with it – this included therapy.

It turns out that I, like many people, especially women, had somehow in my childhood assimilated the message that I should always stay in control. Losing control would mean making a public spectacle of myself, which would be a huge embarrassment to my parents and thus myself.

Years later feminism added another layer to my childhood fear. There was no way that I, as a gender activist, would ever give men the joy of seeing me lose physical or emotional control.

With the birth of superwoman in my early twenties, doing everything perfectly also meant never showing physical weakness.

In one of her Ted Talks[19], Brené Brown quotes the words of an advertisement for Enjoli (a perfume): *"I can put the washing on the line, pack the lunches, hand out the kisses and be at work at five to nine. I can bring home the bacon, fry it up in the pan and never let you forget you're a man."*

Brené said that her research proved that women feel that they "have to do it all, do it perfectly and never let them see you sweat." When women "fail", they are hit by what she calls a "shame shitstorm."

The irony is, of course, that it is an impossibly high standard to meet. Everyone would "fail" at some stage. Unsurprisingly, for me it often materialised through my body. I always wanted to do it all, while not letting anyone

---

[19] https://www.ted.com/talks/brene_brown_listening_to_shame?utm_sourc e=tedcomshare&utm_medium=social&utm_campaign=tedspread

see the proverbial – and with menopause, literal – sweat. If I thought that anyone spotted the "sweat marks", I would find myself in a shame spiral and just worked harder.

For almost five decades, I slept far less than I should, because I didn't have enough hours in the day to be the perfect MP, ambassador, mum, wife and housewife. I pushed through the resulting exhaustion and when pain and illness came, I would take medication (or not) and tell myself to toughen up. I hid my vertigo behind avoidance and false excuses, all in an attempt to not feel the shame my physical vulnerability inflicted on me.

When I finally understood all of this I wanted to cry. I felt a deep sadness for the pressure I had always put myself through.

I also realised that in the darkness of silence, the shame and fear grew more and more. "If you put shame in a petri dish it needs three things to grow exponentially: secrecy, silence and judgement," says Brené.

"How do I fix this?" I ask Abraham.

"You have to silence the voice of the audience," he says. "Those who you think will judge, laugh at and criticize you."

In a professional capacity I have done that for years. I'm not on social media. I believe that social media makes arseholes of just about everyone who's on it. I seldom read the comments below my weekly online newspaper column and on the rare occasion that I do, I know it's a big mistake. I have a small group of people that I trust and whose feedback I value, but I agree with Brené Brown when she says: "If you are not in the arena getting your ass kicked on occasion, I am not interested in or open to your feedback. There are a million cheap seats in the world today filled with people who will never be brave with their own lives but will spend every ounce of energy they have hurling advice and judgement at those of us trying to dare greatly. Their only contributions are criticism, cynicism, and fearmongering. If you're criticizing from a place where you're not also putting yourself on the line, I'm not interested in your feedback."[20]

Of course, I also had to admit that the far more damaging and insidious voice was my own inner critic. She was the one causing all the fear and anxiety.

"You have to feel good about yourself," continued Abraham. "You have to be empathetic to yourself." (I remembered that Brené called empathy the antidote for shame.)

"And" continued Abraham, "while you are busy with this process, you have to know where you are fragile. The chicken will come out of the egg, but not if the egg is cracked too early. Know your boundaries. It is ok to say no."

---

[20] https://www.goodreads.com/quotes/9855106-if-you-are-not-in-the-arena-getting-your-ass

There was the self-love of the vision board workshop again.

Months later during my visit to Ireland, I asked my friend Brid, who is a phenomenal body worker and healer, how she felt I could heal.

She thought about it and the answered firmly: "You will heal when you write about it." Her response surprised me, but on reflection, I knew she was right. Putting it on paper would, after all, ensure that the petri-dish of shame would no longer be fed by silence, secrecy and judgement.

I also knew that I had to do a lot of physical work. I had done extensive physiotherapy after the operation. After two months, I went back to working with my trusted Pilates instructor. I also started to swim.

It all helped, but my body still felt alien to me.

While giving me a massage, Brid, remarked on how much sadness I still seemed to hold in my body. "It is all around your lower abdomen," she said. I told her that I felt so much grief about the organs that were removed and just kept on wondering what was there now.

"Is it just a void?" I asked.

"You have to energetically put it back," she responded. "The energy of your uterus, ovaries and cervix is still available to you, but you have to allow it back."

She then helped me to visualize the organs that were

removed and to see them in a light pink light of energy back in my abdomen.

Weeks later after my return home, I decided to go to an osteopath. Years earlier I had found great relief from osteopathy and hoped that this would help me again with the vertigo.

My journey with Erwann, a French osteopath who is also a doula, was – and continues to be – an extraordinary experience. His deeply empathetic nature and gentle body work was exactly what I needed at the time. He not only did the hands-on work, but also engaged me on an intellectual and intuitive level.

By that stage, I had started to wonder if the vertigo was part of a bigger issue. Yes, pressure from my neck did cause dizziness – but I had only on very rare occasions become so dizzy that I could no longer sit up – so actually it was more a case of being anxious about the anxiety than the physical issue.

I had also started to wonder if the dizziness and heart palpitations that I had experienced since the onset of menopause could be signposts for me. "Could they be trying to tell me something about what I should be doing or not doing?" I asked Erwann.

He nodded.

"It is all one," he said quietly.

I suddenly remembered reading how the author Sue-

Monk Kidd suffered from dangerously high blood pressure in her early fifties. In *Travelling with Pomegranates*, she relates how – despite taking medication – her daily readings would remain high.

At the time she was struggling with the idea of writing a novel. She was resisting it, since it felt too much of a radical departure from the normal Christian writing that she was known for. So, she continued to dismiss the consistent nudge she felt to write a story about bees.

Eventually she gave in and wrote *The Secret Life of Bees*, which went on to be a huge success. During that time her blood pressure problem miraculously disappeared.

Could these episodes of vertigo and heart palpitations be my psyche telling me that I needed to change things?

During the two weeks in Wales when I devoted my time to writing, I had no vertigo. Whilst at the monastery, when I was miserable, the vertigo and palpitations were a daily struggle. They also seemed to be more pronounced when I did political analysis.

I believed there was at least some truth in what he was saying, but also knew that it would take time to figure out what form the change should take.

In the meantime, I knew that at the least I had to change the way I thought about my body. For far too long, I had thought of her as broken and not reliable.

I started to do daily affirmations – affirming that my body

was 100% healthy, strong and beautiful. I also affirmed that I trusted, respected and honoured her. Over time, it certainly helped to change some of my negative thought patterns.

I also had to become aware of the fact that I seemed always to be physically and mentally preparing for some catastrophe. I'm not sure exactly where that came from, but it began when I was very young and became much worse after the operation.

It was a lot, but it was not all of it. I also had to grapple with thoughts of aging and death.

Aging

If the doctors are to be believed, I grew old in the week that I turned fifty. That week I had a doctor's appointment. There was no mention of my age and I was given a prescription and some supplements. A week later I returned for a follow-up visit. The doctor frowned at my file and suggested a series of tests. I was feeling better, so I wanted to know why. "Well, at your age, one should be extra careful."

It seems that fifty is when one enters the "at your age" stage of life. Just like that! One day you are still young and the next day you are at "that age" where things are expected to start breaking down. A bit like when a car reaches 100,000 km and you start to expect things to go wrong – not the oil and brake pad type of things, but the "mechanic shaking his head" type of breakdowns.

I, of course, felt no different.

To be honest, I did feel a little anxious in the run-up to the big 5-0, not because I was feeling older, but because I was worried that I would start *thinking* of myself as old. It was my head and not my body that I was concerned about.

However, after a lovely birthday, life continued and I still felt and thought of myself as young and vibrant.

It was four years later, a month after my 54th birthday, that the gynae shook her head like a car mechanic... and the wheels came off. I was shocked at the ease with which a hysterectomy was mentioned. I didn't want a hysterectomy. I knew it was a very big operation, but more to the point, it felt to me that it was an old woman's operation.

"Why are you so against it?" asked specialist after specialist. "You don't need the organs anymore." Medically speaking, they were right: even if I wanted to have more babies – which I didn't – that ship had sailed.

The day the tumour was discovered was exactly a year after my last period, and coincidentally, 31 years after my first baby was born, so I was officially post-menopausal.

The previous few years were challenging as my hormones started to jump around and eventually flickered into non-existence, and because I get very bad reactions to any hormonal treatment, I had to go through it cold turkey.

It was not fun, and it annoyed me that there were so few discussions acknowledging the impact this process had on women's minds and bodies. In almost all western societies we now talk freely about sex and menstruation. However, menopause is still rarely discussed, even amongst women. To make matters worse, very few doctors are trained in how to manage menopause.

Like most women, I suffered in silence and just got on with it. "Superwoman" was certainly not going to admit to the men in the boardroom that she was having menopausal symptoms, even as the sweat of a hot flush poured down her back during a presentation.

At one big investment seminar, I ran into a woman who was frantically fanning herself in the restroom. "Hot flush?" I asked. She nodded. "I call it a power surge," she responded. I liked that.

The hot flushes interrupted sleep, and other physical symptoms were uncomfortable, but what I hated most were the emotional and brain changes. I need to be super sharp in my work and I experienced huge shame and panic when, out of the blue, I would experience these mental blanks – or as a friend calls it CRAFT (can't remember a fucking thing) moments.

I even worried that it was early onset dementia, but as with all the other symptoms, it turned out to be a perfectly normal "at your age" thing.

"THEN WHY DO WE NOT TALK ABOUT THIS MORE?" I wanted to shout. Instead, millions of women go through this debilitating change alone, filled with fear and shame.

At the same time, women also have to deal with double standards when it comes to aging. Older men in our society are revered for wisdom and experience. I know men who go to hairdressers once a month to cover their grey hair, only to then add grey highlights because it makes them look wiser!

In contrast, very few cultures honour or celebrate middle and older aged women. The comedian Jenny Éclair says that women of a certain age are not only invisible, but get ignored – like not being served at a bar with younger clientele or being forgotten in a clothing room by a sales lady who was getting a bigger size[21] (true stories).

There are a lot of questions as to why this happens.

The media certainly doesn't help. Even though there have been some amazing films starring older women, they are usually portrayed as the grumpy or friendly granny. Or they appear in advertisements for aged-linked medication.

Jenny Éclair again: "The media don't really like ageing women. We are not attractive. There's a lot of deep-rooted misogyny that hovers around like a bad smell. It is not as public as it used to be, but it still lingers. We are dismissed."

I believe that this has a lot to do with a subconscious belief that once women are no longer of child-bearing age, their role in society becomes negligible.

The irony is that if women can get over or manage the difficulties of menopause, they usually look forward to a second phase of their lives. Finally, free of childbearing and rearing responsibilities, they are ready to take on the world.

Christiane Northrup[22], in her book *The Wisdom of Menopause,* says this is why many marriages end in divorce during the middle age years. According to her,

---

[21] https://www.belfasttelegraph.co.uk/life/weekend/jenny-middle-aged-women-arent-invisible-theyre-just-ignored-39391761.html
[22] Christiane Northrup. *The wisdom of menopause.* Philips, 2021 P10

men often start to think about retiring and taking things slower just when women are raring to go back into the labour market.

As women get older, there is also a change in how they are perceived by others and themselves in relation to sexuality.

Czech-born super model Paulina Porizkova said that around the age of 45 she became aware that she was perceived differently from what she was used to. She would post photos of herself in bikinis and the comments were vicious: "Are you a little desperate, grandma? How about you cover up and spare us the look of your poor, aging body?"[23]

Paulina, now fifty-six and still stunningly beautiful, said that this really fired her up, because she thought: "Oh no no no no no, you don't get to tell me how I should perceive myself."

As people age, there is also a massive difference in attitude toward male sexuality versus female sexuality. Older men are usually thought of as virile and sexually active. The opposite is true for women.

I once looked up the female version of "virile". The only word that Google could come up was "muliēbris". I had never heard that word before. On investigation, Wiktionary explained that "*Muliēbris* is derived from *mulier* (woman; wife) (from *mollior* (softer; milder;

---

[23] https://fb.watch/eeiOBZUB9S/

weaker), comparative form of *mollis* (soft; mild, tender; weak), ultimately from Proto-Indo-European **mel-* ("soft; tender; weak")) + *-brīs* (*noun suffix denoting a person*)."[24]

Go figure.

"Muliēbris" aside, while men remain virile, older women are often seen as dried up or asexual after menopause.

Of course, women themselves often have to confront their own sexual histories and wounds. The same was true for me as I tried to deal with my changing body before, and especially after, the operation.

Religion entered my life early. We went to church every Sunday and after the hour-long service there was another hour of Sunday School. During the week there was also "kinderkrans" – Bible study for little children, at someone's house.

When puberty hit, the church made it very clear that sex was to be resisted at all cost. In particular, it was the woman's job to save the men from their evil sexual temptations. Apparently, from the time of Adam and Eve it was always women who seduced men and caused their fall from grace.

I bought it... and during my teenage years doubled up on church attendance and Bible study. I also didn't drink, smoke or dance (I figured it was best to resist all temptations). Any boyfriends were strictly limited to

---

[24] https://en.wiktionary.org/wiki/muliebrity

kissing and handholding. Despite that, I was once berated by a church councillor for wearing white jeans during a camp. Apparently, that was irresistible to boys and I was therefore committing a very serious sin.

This message remained ever present as I studied theology at university in the hope of becoming a minister in the church. Three years later, at the age of 20, I married Wilhelm.

I was often asked by friends why we got married so early.

The honest answer was that we wanted to have sex and were petrified that we might "fall" if we had to wait much longer. Unsurprisingly, the honeymoon turned out to be a disaster.

It wasn't fun, and there were no fireworks. We were married for 19 years and as time went on, my husband's reaction convinced me that I was just not good at it. As the state of our marriage got worse, the sex also got worse, which I assumed was my fault. (Or was it that the marriage got worse because sex got worse?)

By the time of the divorce, I had zero sexual confidence left. I had internalised the explicit and implicit messages that I was hopeless in bed.

There was also a bigger issue at stake. From early in my teenage years, I hated the way men and boys would talk about women's bodies. I realised quickly that they not only thought of women as dangerous seductresses, but believed that women's bodies were there for their pleasure.

I really abhorred – and still do – the fact that so many men use sexuality to belittle and disempower women through language (jokes), body language (leering) and far too often fear (threat of sexual violence).

Of course, I was well aware that sexuality could be a powerful tool for women too: to be used for professional advancement or to gain material benefit. Yet, even as a very young girl, I knew that there was a price to pay. I knew, intuitively, that using sexuality in that way meant giving up freedom, especially the freedom to lay claim and ownership to your own body.

I was always very clear that my body belonged to me, at least in the public domain. I would hide behind short boyish haircuts and had (as a therapist later described it) a general "Fuck off" attitude as far as men were concerned.

The problem was that I bought my own story and started to believe that I was unattractive, and this added to the woes in my marriage. It was only when I met Gerry – many years after my divorce – that I discovered the real joy of physical intimacy. Through positive feedback and laughter, I gradually started to heal. I also started to embrace my feminine side – growing my hair and wearing clothes that really made me feel good about myself.

This did not change as I got "older", but the hysterectomy threw me. After the initial healing process, my body felt different. Despite the doctor's reassurance, I was nervous about getting hurt and wondered in particular about the stitches where the cervix used to be. Also, the final bowing out of oestrogen changed my desires.

Building a new relationship with my body and sexuality is an ongoing journey of gentle discovery, but there are a few things that I know now for sure:

Women are as much sexual beings as men, but only if we are willing to claim that truth and get over the goodgirl messages we have been indoctrinated with since childhood.

I'm also very clear that my body and sexuality belong to me and not to anyone else. My body and sexuality are primarily for my enjoyment and not for that of any man. Therefore, if a man is interested in his own pleasure only – as so many men are – I have no interest in being with him.

Of course, I cannot deny that the body starts to change with time and these changes are not always fun – as Nora Ephron so hilariously describes in her book, *I feel bad about my neck.* For example, she writes about her annoyance with people who say that it is great to be old – to be "wise and sage and mellow" and to understand what matters in life. "I can't stand people who say things like this," says Ephron. "What can they be thinking? Don't they have necks? She claims that one of her biggest regrets in life is that she did not spend her youth staring lovingly at her neck. "It never crossed my mind to be grateful for it," she says. "Of course, it's true that now that I'm older, I'm wise and sage and mellow. And it is also true that I

honestly do understand just what matters in life. But guess what? It's my neck. [25]
In the social media world of eternal youth, it is difficult to deal with these changes. Still, we should not only accept but celebrate them. As Michelle Obama, who of course looks like she is still 30 years old, said to Oprah: "At 56, this body cannot do what it did at 36. It is not the same body."

She is right!

Our bodies are living things that change. As Michelle rightly points out: to expect to look at 55 as one did at 37, or to be judged for not looking the same, is as ridiculous as expecting to still fit into clothes that one wore at the age of ten.[26]

It takes a lot of work to feel confident in our (especially uncovered) bodies as we grow older. Part of the reason is that the world tells us that to be attractive we need to look wrinkle free, skinny and without a grey hair in sight.

I am fully aware that I'm not free of these myths, but I am working hard to liberate myself. A while ago I decided to surround myself with images of women who do not meet the stereotypically emaciated, tall, big breasted, botoxed images that we in the West are told personifies beauty.

On my desk I have a row of photos: The first one is of my friend Nadine from Jamaica, who is one of the most

---

[25] Nora Ephron: *I feel bad about my neck.* Black Swan, 2006
[26] https://www.youtube.com/watch?v=XvFaaO5b4hE

beautiful women I know. On the photo she stands in a bathing suit in the ocean, her head thrown back. In her mid-fifties, she is muscled from years of exercise and radiates strength and beauty.

I also have a photo of P!nk on a trapeze at one of her shows. She is wearing a leotard with her powerful thighs and arms exposed – her strength, sexuality and beauty undeniable.

Next to P!nk is Alicia Keyes without make-up. Her natural inner beauty makes me gasp every time I look at her.

I also have a photo of Bebe Vio, the Olympic gold medallist in fencing. She lost both her arms and legs and has deep scars on her face after contracting meningitis at the age of 11. In the photo she is dressed in a beautiful evening gown. With her sabre under her one upper arm (her arms were amputated from just below the elbow) and the fencing mask under the other, she looks into the camera lens with strength and poise.

For me these women embody true beauty and sexuality.

I have also realised how important it is to retain a sense of humour as the body starts changing. Nora Ephron's *I feel bad about my neck* had me in stitches because I recognised some of myself in her writing.

Maya Angelou is another role model for me. On the occasion of her 70th birthday she recited this very funny poem she wrote, named "Don't break the elastic" [27].

When I was in my younger days,
I weighed a few pounds less,
I needn't hold my tummy in
to wear a belted dress.
But now that I am older,
I've set my body free;
There's the comfort of elastic
Where once my waist would be.
Inventor of those high-heeled shoes
My feet have not forgiven;
I have to wear a nine now,
But used to wear a seven.
And how about those pantyhose-
They're sized by weight, you see,
So how come when I put them on
The crotch is at my knee?
I need to wear these glasses
As the print's been getting smaller;
And it wasn't very long ago
I know that I was taller.
Though my hair has turned to grey
and my skin no longer fits,
On the inside, I'm the same old me,
It's the outside's changed a bit.

---

[27] https://atelim.com/in-april-maya-angelou-was-interviewed-by-oprah-on-her-70-birth.html

Brilliant!

Another thing I know is that accepting and even welcoming growing older does not mean giving up. I will continue to eat well and avoid drinking and smoking. Looking after my body will remain important and might take more time and resources as time go by.

I have also realised how vital it is to have a sympathetic, preferably female doctor and other alternative health care professionals, who will work with me to stay in optimal health and prevent disease as much as possible.

I will, of course, continue to do the necessary screenings to catch some of the common diseases as early as possible. However, I no longer want to do it out of fear. Too many healthy-living, anti-aging books are fundamentally fear driven. More often than not they insist on an impossible list of do's and don'ts to prevent an early death from some horrible, but – according to them – perfectly preventable disease.

This takes too much joy out of life. I think Maya Angelou has the right approach when she says: "Do everything in moderation – even moderation."[28]

Ultimately, I think that how we age depends a lot on our state of mind. Next to my beauty role models, I also have photos of Maya herself, David Attenborough and Jane Goodall.

---

[28] https://www.youtube.com/watch?v=SlzrYiKxWdY

Even in his 90's, David Attenborough remains the voice of conscience when it comes to the environment. Jane Goodall at 83 still travels 300 days a year to raise awareness for her foundation. Maya Angelou was 86 and still active when she died.

All of them have always, and in the cases of Attenborough and Goodall, still do, work harder than most people. Perhaps this is helped by good genetics, but I strongly believe that the fact that they pursue causes that they feel passionate about, and which are bigger than themselves, is largely the reason for their age defying looks and lifestyle.

They share a joyful curiosity in everything around them. Perhaps Brené Brown is right when she says that curiosity is the superpower of the second part of our lives.[29]

I have warned my children that I'm planning to live until I'm at least 105. I hope that I will get to that age.

Perhaps I won't, but in the meantime, I will try to embrace the changes aging will bring in my body and my soul. Like the three non-aging heroes on my desk, I will look at life with curiosity while doing something meaningful, and always expecting deep joy.

And I will look forward to every decade as it comes.

To return to Maya Angelou: when asked by Oprah what she could say about being in her 80's after she was so

---

[29] https://www.youtube.com/watch?v=6j7DbxtMbpQ

excited about being 60 and 70, she responded:

"Oh, my goodness! Do it if you can! If you have a choice, choose the 80's. I mean it!"

Death

The night before the operation I was lying awake in the dark. Images of myself on the theatre table haunted me. "I might die tomorrow," I suddenly thought.

Strangely enough it didn't scare me.

I have never had any doubts that we keep on existing in some form after death. It is not that I believe in heaven and hell as physical spaces, but I do believe that we continue in some different energetic form.

Shortly after Gerry's passing, a book agent in Ireland suggested that I go and see a medium. "Look, unlike most Irish people, I don't believe in that stuff," she said. "But Paddy McMahon is amazing." She passed me his book, *Guided by Angles: There are No Goodbyes.*[30] Over the next few nights I read his life story. I was doubtful, but so distraught that I decided to contact him.

To me it was clear as daylight that Gerry's big energy couldn't just have disappeared. How could he just be gone? Where is gone? Even quantum physics tells us that energy never disappears, it only changes form. So perhaps Paddy could help.

Paddy lived in a nondescript house in a housing estate on the outskirts of Dublin. After greeting me warmly at the

---

[30] Paddy McMahon. *Guided by Angles: There are no Goodbyes.* Collins. 2011

door, he explained that on account of his advanced age he rarely did these sessions anymore, but when I called, he felt compelled to say yes. "I'm a little nervous," he confided. "Please know I can't always connect. Sometimes the departed don't want to communicate."

"Well, if anyone would love to talk – it would be Gerry," I joked lamely, attempting to hide my own nervousness.

Over the next few hours, I had the most extraordinary experience of my life. Paddy channelled Gerry and relayed things that only Gerry and I knew. It blew my mind. When I left, I was exhausted, but felt strangely comforted.

Over the years, I have continued to feel Gerry's, and my beloved maternal grandmother's presence. I don't particularly care if it is real or imagined – all I know is that it helps me.

On the night before the operation, I got up, took my will out of the filing cabinet and put it on the corner of my desk where my children would easily spot it.

Then I thought about dying. I truly felt at peace about the idea of dying on the operating table. I was confident I would connect with Gerry again – and that would be fantastic. However, I didn't want a long painful death. I did *not* want cancer.

I also knew that my death would be devastating for my children and that alone was a good enough reason to want to hang around a bit longer. Earlier, I had asked friends around the world to keep me in their thoughts while I was on the operating table. Now I called on Gerry and my grandmother to be in the theatre with me too.

In the seconds before the anaesthetic took effect, I thought of my grandmother and Gerry hovering in the theatre and Nadine in Jamaica, Malcolm in New Zealand, Brid in Dublin and my family and friends in South Africa – all holding me in a big global embrace.

... And I didn't die.

Not yet anyway...

But... I will die because, annoyingly, we all die.

After the operation, I started to think a lot about death. I could no longer postpone it for when I was old. I had come too close...

It was not that death hadn't touched my life. Two decades earlier, I had lost my beloved grandfather and grandmother in quick succession. My two dads, Bennie and Philip, had died – albeit three decades apart. Then of course there was the almost unbearable loss of Gerry. We had also just gone through COVID where death seemed to be a constant companion.

Still, facing my own death was very different.

I had wondered why this operation had thrown me so much. A few years earlier, I had surgery to remove a lump in my breast. A decade before, that a strange bubble appeared on my one eye. In both cases, they turned out to be benign.

Still, unlike with the other two incidents, this one had shaken me to the core.

A few weeks after the operation, I watched a movie called "The Professor". Richard, played by Johnny Depp, declines treatment for terminal lung cancer and is given six months to live. In the weeks that follow, he re-evaluates his life and what is important to him.

At what turns out to be his final faculty dinner party, he says: "We have to make death our closest companion so that we can finally have a milli-second to appreciate what little time we have left."

I realised that this is what had happened to me. For the two weeks before my operation and a few days after, death was my constant companion. Having to look my own death in the eye for the first time rewired me. Even though the tumour turned out to be benign, I knew that my life would forever be divided into a time before the operation and a time after.

Jean Shinoda Bolen in her book *Close to the Bone: Life-threatening Illness as a Soul Journey* says: "When death becomes close, soul questions arise."[31]

I had faced the possibility of serious, potentially deadly

---

[31] Jean Shinoda Bolen. *Close to the bone: Life-threatening Illness as a Soul Journey*. Conari Press. 2007.

illness and unsurprisingly my soul was now asking many questions. In particularly, she wanted me to evaluate the way I conducted my life and to clarify what was most important to me going forward.

A free woman

"It was the first decision I took as a free woman."

My eyes lingered over the short sentence. I had read *Untamed* by Glennon Doyle a few times, but had never really focused on this sentence. Until now.

"A free woman, a free woman…"

I rolled the words around in my head.

"What does it mean to be truly free? What would it take to be totally free? What would it look like for me to be a truly free woman?"

I knew that these were the questions that I had been struggling with my whole life.

Of course, central to all freedom are the basic human rights that all people are entitled to. I grew up in a country where the majority of people were denied the most basic of freedoms - of speech, association and physical safety. I spent most of my adult life fighting for these freedoms to be restored in South Africa.

However, even though these rights are undeniably crucial, they were not the freedoms that I was searching for on my journey of recovery.

I was yearning for the freedom of my soul.

Deep in our souls and bodies we all carry the wounds and fears of a lifetime of living. Some of these wounds are so debilitating that we cannot ignore them. Others are more insidious and, like dangerous parasites, they exhaust us, often without our even knowing what is holding us back from the life of inner freedom we long for.

Following the operation, I started to deal with so many of these fear parasites. It was not easy – in fact it was almost as painful as the surgery. There is something extremely uncomfortable about acknowledging, naming and understanding our fears. It creates vulnerability and shame.

My battle with these fear-provoking demons was long overdue, yet none the less very scary. I came to realise that many of my wounds and fears were mechanisms to create a sense of safety, but that this "safety net" was full of huge holes and that, rather than protecting me, it was suffocating me. The truth was that these fears no longer served me and possibly never had.

So, in order to be truly free, I had to go into battle against goodgirl, superwoman and bag lady. I had to look aging and death in the eye. I had to befriend and trust my body. I also had to deal with the deep painful wounds left by my dad and my goodbyes to the men that I truly loved.

I also had to accept that these battles are never completely won. As with the aftermath of a big bush fire, there would always be embers waiting to ignite. For the rest of my life, I would have to stay alert and spot the smoke early.

"One has to distinguish between freedoms from... and freedoms to..." said one of my fellow writers one night in Wales. I know she is right.

As much relief as facing these fears gave me, I knew that was only half of the story. Perhaps I was free, or at least freer, from them, but what now?

There was still "the freedom to..." part. What were these inner freedoms that I wanted to claim?

A few days later I read a story about Alicia Keyes. In 2016 the multi-award-winning singer, announced that she would no longer wear make-up. She explained that she had come to realise that she was dependent on cosmetics to feel confident and didn't want that. What a bombshell, in the Hollywood world of false eyelashes and heavy foundation!

A while later, she was one of the judges on the TV show, *The Voice*. One of her fellow judges, Adam Levine, tells of how he popped into her dressing room one day and saw her putting on lipstick.

"Hey," he said, "I thought you don't wear make-up?"

Alicia turned around slowly in her chair, locked eyes with him and said quietly: "I do whatever the fuck I want!"

I do whatever the fuck I want!

When I read that story, it nearly took my breath away. I whispered the words repeatedly to myself. I knew I wanted to make that my battle cry! I wanted to embrace the vast freedom that statement promised. Just to think about it made my body shiver and my head dizzy.

That night I wrote down the battle cry for the next part of my life in my diary:

> *I will do what I want.*
> *I will wear what I want.*
> *I will weigh what I want.*
> *I will feel and show the emotions I want.*
> *I will say what I want.*
> *I will be with who I want, if I want.*
> *I will turn up fully – as me.*
> *I will insist to be seen and be heard.*
> *I WILL belong to myself.*

I felt enormous liberation. Of course, I knew that it did not come without responsibilities and boundaries. I needed to position this within a framework of values that are important to me, of which kindness was the most important.

I have always believed that if kindness was at the centre of every action and decision we take, the world would be a much better place. So, to be truly free to feel, say and do what I want, I cannot be unkind to others.

Kindness had to remain my beacon in all that I did.

It also meant being kind to myself. So, I had to keep my body healthy and fit, by eating well and doing exercise. I had to continue with my spiritual practice, for which I needed silence and retreat. I had to rest frequently and above all, work at a pace that allowed my body and soul to breathe.

Ultimately, it means that while I may be willing to sacrifice and even suffer for the benefit of others, I must never do it in ways that violate the essence of who I am.

Having written my battle cry was empowering... for a short while

Then it hit me: It was fine to say that I would do and say what I wanted, but what did I want to do and say?

As is often the case, it was far easier to know what I didn't want, than to figure out what I really, really wanted. (Sorry, I had to bring in the Spice Girls at some point!)

I knew it had something to do with what gave me joy. After all, what was freedom without joy?

This reminded me of my wetsuit expedition of few months earlier.

Finding joy

I stared at the black rubber thing on my bed with trepidation.

What if I couldn't get out of it again? What if I had to call someone to come and cut me loose? How long would it take for them to get here? How embarrassing would that be?"

I felt a hot flush starting.

"Would sweating make it worse?"

Earlier that day I had bought a wet suit. In the weeks after my operation, I kept thinking that being in the ocean would help my physical and more importantly, emotional healing.

I love the ocean and with the exception of the first five years of my life, as well as two years in the UK, I have always lived close to the sea. As a teenager I would run into the ocean at any opportunity – irrespective of the weather.

For some reason I stopped doing that years... ok, who am I kidding... decades ago.

I blame the cold... and Ireland.

The Irish have a habit of jumping into the freezing sea irrespective of the weather – but to me that is certifiable craziness. Even for someone who grew up next to the South Atlantic, the cold was unbearable.

So, when I went to Ireland, I stopped going into the ocean, opting for walks next to it instead.

Even after my return to South Africa I never found my sea mojo again.

A few weeks after the operation, while watching my retrievers frolicking with joyful abandonment in the waves, I felt a strong sense of longing to get back in. I wanted to feel the power of the waves and the exhilarating combination of salt, sun and sand on my skin.

"I'm thinking of buying a wetsuit," I WhatsApped my son – who loves surfing – in Dublin.

Long pause.

Him: "Eh WHY?"

Me: "I want to get into the ocean."

Longer pause.

Him: "Eh WHY?"

Me: "I want to swim and it's cold."

Even longer pause.

Him: "Oooh... keey."

Me: "Any advice?"

Him: "Go to a shop and try some on."

Me: "Smart arse!"

He sent me links to a few outlet shops – clearly not convinced about the longevity of my newest endeavour.

The idea of going to a shop with hundreds of wetsuits didn't appeal to me. It wasn't so much the wetsuits, but rather the idea of having to ask some gorgeous, tanned twenty-something with sun bleached hair to help me squeeze into a few different wetsuits, whilst trying to ignore the thinly veiled "gosh-she-is-so-old" look.

Clearly, that would have defeated the purpose of rediscovering my youthful self, so I dropped the idea.

To complicate matters, I had just finished reading *Let My People Go Surfing* by Yvon Chouinard, the founder and head of the outdoor company, Patagonia. Until that point, I had never known how damaging Neoprene, the material most wetsuits are made of, is for the environment. I thought about buying one of Patagonia's sustainably sourced rubber suits, but it cost nearly four times the price of other suits and that seemed a bit excessive – especially since my son's scepticism might prove to be valid.

So, I turned to my new secret pleasure: Facebook Marketplace.

For decades I had resisted all attempts by family, friends

and business associates to lure me into joining Facebook. As already mentioned, I think that social media makes even the nicest people arseholes, and since I didn't want to become an arsehole, I had stayed away.

Then I discovered Facebook Marketplace.

The catch was that to get the key to this wonderous world of peer-to-peer trading – the fancy name for it according to my daughter - where you could buy anything for a steal, I had to first get a Facebook profile.

Bummer!

I eventually got my PA to create a Facebook profile for me – where apparently hundreds of people who I had never met, and never intend to meet, befriended me within weeks. I say "apparently" because I have never looked at it. Over the last few months, I have only clicked on the little house icon at the bottom of the screen and spent far too much time wondering where I could place a purple couch or a red carpet.

It turned out that there was a seemingly endless supply of second-hand wetsuits available in my area – mostly "condition as new – barely used." I knew my son would make a "yes-all-those-middle-aged-women-who-thought-they-wanted-to-go-swimming" sound at that.

A Rip Curl, size 12, tags still attached, caught my eye. But would it fit?

I googled the Rip Curl size chart. It looked a bit small – especially over my newly operated stomach.

I WhatsApped my son the pictures.

Me: "What do you think?"

Him: "Looks a bit long, no?"

Me: "I'm more worried about it being too tight."

Him: "It must be tight, otherwise it doesn't work, but also not too tight – then you won't be able to breathe."

Me: "How would I know?"

Him: "Go to the shops and try some on."

SIGH!

I decided against the purchase but over the next few weeks the suit kept popping up as good old Facebook cleverly read my mind.

"Should I just go and try it on at seller5063's house?" I wondered.

Deciding that it was even worse than the shop filled with the sun bleached blonde haired twenty-year old assistants, I abandoned the idea.

Instead, I made a low offer for the suit. I reasoned that

if it was too small, I would give it to my sister, who has annoyingly shown no sign of any middle age flab.

The offer was accepted, and I collected it.

A few hours later, I stared anxiously at the wetsuit lying on my bed.

My son and brother-in-law had entertained us once with stories of getting stuck in their wetsuits and having panic attacks as they waited for help. I had nightmares about suffocating in my clothes afterwards and now they all came back.

"Shall I risk it?" I asked my two retrievers, who were lying next to the bed. They started to pant – which is apparently a sign of stress.

I WhatsApped my daughter who lives a few houses away.

"Trying on a wetsuit. If you get a missed call – come over quickly and bring scissors."

She "LOL"-ed back.

I put my phone within easy reach, then pulled and hopped and squeezed.

Sweating and panting faster than my retrievers, I finally popped the second shoulder in, held my breath and pulled up the zip.

I was in!

I looked in the mirror.

Ok, there was a feint resemblance to the Michelin man – but I could live with it.

Now the big test.

The retrievers gave anxious yawns and left the room.

Ten minutes later, after a lot more huffing, puffing, hopping, twisting and some swearing, I sat sweating on the side of the bed, with the wetsuit at my feet.

VICTORY!!

Two days later I stood next to the ocean, watching my dogs riding the waves with their big retriever smiles.

The yearning was back.

It was now or never.

I ran back to the house where I was staying, slipped on my bathing costume and hopped and squeezed again into the wetsuit. I asked my friend to keep an eye on me from his balcony, in case I fainted from oxygen deprivation, which could apparently happen with too tight a wetsuit. My friend's deep-sea-diver son had "helpfully" shared this information with me the previous night.

I strolled over the beach and slowly walked into the water. My feet were freezing, but my legs felt fine.

I took a deep breath and dived into the water...

I remembered!

For 20 minutes, I blissfully bopped around in the water like a black Teletubby – giggling at the buoyancy the wetsuit gave me.

Back on dry land, I pulled the suit off my shoulders and down to my waist.

As I strolled back to the house, I laughed out loud.

I felt stronger and more alive than I had for years. Hell, I felt like a 20-year-old with sun bleached hair!

"Are you going to swim to the other side of the bay?" asked a woman, walking her dogs.

"Not today..." I replied.

Months later, I thought again about the experience.

Perhaps the key to unlocking this deep sense of freedom I had been craving for most of my life lay in finding joy. Not a superficial type of happiness, but a joy that lies deep in my cells and makes them jiggle like jelly on a plate.

In *Runaway Bride*, Julia Roberts' character realises that she has never figured out what type of eggs she likes because she has always made and ordered them the way her various partners have wanted them. I knew exactly how I liked my eggs (totally dead), but when it came to a lot of other things, I would often compromise because of financial prudence, the approval of others, or just so I wouldn't stand out. More often than not, I simply didn't make time to determine what truly mattered to me because it seemed like a terrible luxury or indulgence.

It was time to figure out how I liked my proverbial eggs.

I made long lists of things I liked, and even longer lists of things I didn't. I vowed to do more and get more of what I liked whilst abandoning and ridding myself of everything on the dislike list.

After many weeks, I was still restless.

Then, I remembered Marie Kondo.

Years ago, long before she became a world-wide phenomenon. I had bought her book *Sparking Joy*.

Marie, a Japanese organiser, believes that the only reason to have or hold on to something in your life is that it "sparks joy". When decluttering, she insists that you touch every object and ask: "Does it spark joy for me?" If it does, you keep it, if it doesn't, you thank it and let it go. No "what if I may need it?" or "but it was very expensive" is allowed. I was wondering if Marie's method could help me to figure out what I really wanted in life. It had worked for me in my house, could it be helpful with my inner journey?

I had, after all, done some inner decluttering by reducing and hopefully eliminating, but what was holding me back and making me unhappy. Could I now figure out what actually gave me joy?

I knew that it couldn't only be linked to feelings of happiness which can be fleeting – as when having made a pleasing purchase. I was searching for much more so – I kid you not – I googled: "how to know what sparks joy". Helpfully, there was a video of Marie Kondo[32] explaining just that.

Holding onto a piece of clothing, she closed her eyes and breathed in deeply. Then, with a big smile, she pointed a finger into the air and lifted slightly onto her toes. "Chiiiiing!" she said in a high pitch. It immediately made me smile.

"When there is a spark of joy," she explained, "it feels as if every part or cell of your body lifts – little by little. Compare this to the opposite when your body feels heavy and weighs you down."

She then made a deep "Nzeeee" sound.

I immediately understood. The answer lies in the body. It is what Glennon Doyle describes as sinking into the body and why Malcolm had asked me all those weeks ago: "How does that make you feel?"

He wasn't asking me for an emotional response. Instead, he wanted me to check in with my body, because, as he

---

[32] *https://www.youtube.com/watch?v=_ea6i0J8W2U*

often reminds me, the body never lies. Unlike our head and mouth, it can't. It will tell us if we are sick, stressed or in danger. It can also tell us if a situation is right for us, if only we would listen to it.

So, I started to put things through the "Chiiiing" test and to take note of what made every part or cell of my body "lift up".

Naturally for me, spending time with my children and looking forward to my grandchildren were top of the list.

I also knew that nature in general and animals specifically made my body vibrate with joy. Being able to use my voice particularly through my writing, to touch people's hearts and change the world for the better was a big CHIIIIIING! Dancing, "ching". Swimming, "ching". Being in a minimalist space, "ching".

I also made a "Nzeee" list.

Cardio workouts: "Nzeeeeeeeeee;" I've always believed, that if God wanted me to run, she wouldn't have given me breasts. Going out to restaurants or parties: "Nzeee." Public speaking on things I don't care about: big NZEEEEEEE!

In the months to come, in deciding what do and say I sought and listened to my body's response. It worked and I determined to trust my body in future decision-making.

If I felt the "Chiiiing!" I would go for it. "Nzeeee," and I would walk away.

I finally understood that a huge part of achieving freedom was claiming it! Yes, basic freedoms had to be guaranteed in law, but being truly free, was an internal process. It was the acknowledgement and gentle silencing of the inner critic, the inner denier of joy. Yes, these voices often originated from our childhood or traumatic events – like discovering the growth or Gerry's death – but I had a choice. I had to decide whether it was going to "Nzeeee" me for the rest of my life, or whether to let it heal by letting it go.

On my tummy there is a long red scar from the hysterectomy. It serves as a reminder of the place that the surgeons entered my body in order to remove a potentially deadly growth that was crowding out other organs.

I no longer think of it as ugly. It reminds me of the need to be vigilant for the emotional growths that were crowding out joy in my life. It reminds me that every solution, every answer that I seek, lies ultimately within myself.

Above all, it affirms that I truly belong to myself...

And that is utter freedom.

I am here! Finding my voice

There was a famous philosophy professor at the University of Stellenbosch who would start his first lecture to new students with one simple question: "Ladies and gentlemen, ask yourself this: Why were you born at this particular place and time?" Then he paused and left.

That was lecture one done.

I have always understood that my answer to the question was that I was meant to be a voice for justice and in particular for those whose voices went unheard.

Yet, that wasn't always easy. As the only woman in my theology class at university, I was told more than once, that while the powers-that-be could not stop me from being there, the likelihood of me – as a woman – ever being allowed in a pulpit was virtually zero.

However, the first time I really understood the anguish of invisibility was during my marriage. A year after our wedding, Wilhelm and I returned to Oxford in order for him to finish his Rhodes Scholarship. I used the time to research for my Master's thesis – on "God as Mother".

Wilhelm had, over the years, built relations with an organization called Moral Re-Armament – a non-denominational revivalist organization founded after the Second World War. Some of their members had taken Wilhelm under their wing when he first arrived in Europe. They were clearly very impressed with him, his family background and the fact that he was on a Rhodes scholarship.

I, on the other hand, was of very little interest to them. They were friendly and no more sexist than any other organisation, but to them I was only Wilhelm's wife, and at any get together, a mere afterthought, if that.

I deeply resented it.

Years later, after our return to South Africa, I found my voice in politics. Despite all the death threats and personal sacrifices that followed our joining the ANC, I never doubted for a minute that I had done the right thing

Wilhelm was adamant that he was more of a thinker and that I was the activist. So, we made the decision that I would pursue a political career while he stayed in academia. I really loved political work, but Wilhelm began to resent the high-profile nature of my work, and that would eventually play a major part in the eventual breakup of our marriage.

Seven years after I became an MP, it became clear to me that unless I stepped back from the public eye, our marriage would not survive. Hoping that some time abroad would help, I asked the president to appoint me to an ambassadorial posting. He agreed and we went to Ireland.

However, despite moving into reconciliation work, which would change the whole course of his life, Wilhelm's resentment grew. Even though he only accompanied me to two events per year – making my work life very lonely and twice as hard – he didn't appreciate the fact that he was now often seen as "the Ambassador's spouse".

In order to avoid conflict or days of silence, I tried very hard to accommodate him. In social gatherings, I increasingly kept quiet or deferred to him when I was asked questions. It didn't seem to help.

One night, we were invited to a feminist friend of mine's house for dinner. We were joined by two other feminist theologians. The evening was filled with interesting discussions and great food, but I could see Wilhelm brooding and getting into an increasingly dark mood. Feeling the familiar tension rising in me, I made a point of not talking too much. I also tried to pull him into the conversation, by not answering questions I knew he would be interested in. "That's more Wilhelm's field," I would say over and over again.

That night, we drove home in tension-filled silence. Eventually Wilhelm turned to me. "You know that they are not really interested in what you have to say," he said sharply. "They are only being polite because of your position."

It felt like someone had knocked my breath out. Of course, I should have seen it for what it was: our marriage had been over for a while; we were both hurting and Wilhelm was lashing out.

Instead, I tapped into the deep feminine wound that so many women carry, and felt a deep sense of shame. Brené

Brown says that shame is a powerful social tool often used to keep women quiet. "Nothing silences us more effectively than shame."

In that moment, I lost my voice.

For years afterwards – and I still have to watch out for it – I would question myself when telling a story or speaking out. I would often start a story and then stop midway, wondering if people were truly interested. I also became, and still am, fiercely critical of my performance at any public speaking engagement.

Most damaging, I gave up all my dreams of writing.

I was silenced… completely.

More than a decade later, and by then on better terms following the divorce, I reminded Wilhelm of that evening. He looked totally baffled and had no memory of it. Yet, for me, it was deeply damaging.

For years, it felt like I would never find my voice again. Externally I looked powerful. I did my work, but when it came to speaking my truth, the internal question was always there: "What if they are not really interested?"

Eventually, I found the strength to whisper the words: "I need to leave you before I hate you," to my husband. In doing so, the gradual reclamation of my voice began.

In the years after the divorce, I presented radio shows and also became head of UNICEF Ireland – a job I adored.

I found a new love in Gerry and gradually became confident again.

Then Gerry died and because of all the media attention following his death, the Board of UNICEF terminated my contract. Legal action followed and eventually UNICEF settled the case on the precondition that I was not allowed to speak about the settlement or the details of what had happened.

The day I signed the settlement offer at the lawyer's office I wept. It was a good deal, and I really did not want to take UNICEF to court, but I was devastated by the fact that I was being silenced – it felt like a complete and utter betrayal of who I was.

Thankfully I had already published a book[33] which revealed much of what had happened – although on the day of the book launch, there was a court challenge from a former friend of Gerry's to stop its distribution.

An exhausting and expensive legal battle followed, but I was not going to give up. I knew that not publishing the story of my life, my relationship with Gerry and what had happened in UNICEF, would kill me psychologically and possibly even physically.

I eventually agreed to a short clarification in the footnotes and the book became a best seller.

---

[33] The book was first published in Ireland under the title *When We Dance* and later in South Africa as *The Verwoerd who toyi-toyied*.

Nevertheless, I knew I couldn't stay in Ireland much longer. It was clear that because of my relationship with Gerry, I would never be left alone by the media. I would never be able to be my own person again; I would always be seen as "the late Gerry Ryan's girlfriend".

It was then, in 2013, that I went back to South Africa and began the long journey of re-establishing myself again, initially through writing.

I published two more books, this time about other people's stories. After what happened in Ireland, I didn't want to risk the emotional bruising that can come with personal storytelling. Instead, I wrote a book about people who had met Nelson Mandela[34] and then co-authored accounts of young people's experience in the new South Africa[35].

I also built a successful business as a political analyst. Initially, I couldn't believe that people would pay me to talk about politics, but my experience as a member of parliament gave me unique insights that companies valued. I was also invited to write a weekly political column for a large online newspaper.

Somehow, as the years went by, it felt increasingly as if something was still missing. I was writing other people's stories and analysing the political narratives of politicians. I kept it at a distance and didn't let it touch my heart.

---

[34] Melanie Verwoerd. *Our Madiba: Stories and reflections from those who met Nelson Mandela.* NB Publishers 2014

[35] Melanie Verwoerd and Sonwabiso Ngcowa . *"21 @ 21: The coming of age of a nation."* Missing Ink. 2015

Even before the operation, I could feel a gentle nudge to do something new – something more authentically me. The only question was what? Knowing that it might involve difficult and scary decisions, I would push that question to the back of my consciousness.

During the COVID pandemic, I took a deep breath and started to write a few columns from my heart. I loved it, but the editors would remind me that I was there to produce more hardcore political content.

Then came the operation – and the question was no longer a sense of unease or a gentle whisper. It was a loud, urgent voice.

I have no idea what this will mean in practice. What I am certain about, is that I will never be silenced again.

I will also not disappear as I get older.

In the first series of "Grace and Frankie", the two women, played by Jane Fonda and Lily Tomlin, decide to buy cigarettes. Their husbands have just announced that they wish to marry each other, having confessed to a ten-year secret romantic relationship. After the shock, the women decide that they need a "revenge smoke".

At the grocery store, they wait in vain to be served. Seemingly invisible to the young salesman they are first ignored and then overlooked when a young, blonde woman comes to the check-out.

It is at this point that the usually composed Grace loses her cool. "HALLO! HALLO!" she shouts at the top of her voice, while bashing a basket on the counter. "Do you not see me?" she demands of the salesman. "Do I not exist?"

Frankie eventually drags her screaming and yelling out of the store. Back in the car, while Frankie lights a cigarette from the pack she had stolen, Grace says: "Ok, that lacked poise, but I refuse to become irrelevant"

Post-surgery, the words: "I will not become irrelevant, I will not become silent," kept racing through my head.

Having a voice has always been my reason for existence. As much as I wanted to please and be a good girl, I have always known deep inside me that speaking out was why I was in this life and on this earth.

Now, almost a year after the operation, I know that is what I will do for the rest of my life.

I know I have to keep on writing but unlike the many times before, I have to find the courage to do it from my heart. Speaking from the heart and speaking my truth has always been my superpower. When I write columns from my heart it is clear from the comments that the writing touches people deeply – and there's also nothing that give me more joy or "Ching!"

I'm aware that it will often be painful. Writing from my heart requires an opening of the heart, of letting myself be seen warts and all whilst stepping into the arena. This demands a willingness to dive deep into a pool of vulnerability.

It can be brutal, but it is the only way I know to change the world.

The feminist poet Muriel Rukeyser wrote that the world would split open if one woman would tell the truth about her life.

Our world is in desperate need of being "split open". Like Muriel, I know for sure that this will never happen until the voices of women are heard.

I know that these truthful voices threaten the masculine world we live in and that men – and some women – will continue to try and silence us.

Perhaps the biggest gift of my tumour and hysterectomy was that they made me face my own mortality. I had to truly come to terms with the fact that my time on this earth is finite. I had to ask myself what I wanted to do with that time.

I know that I have lost my tolerance for bullshit. I am done with the mundane things which occupy so much time. I want to minimize the clutter of everyday life and fill my days with what is meaningful and fills me with joy.
I am no longer prepared to just "float through this weird thing called life"[36].

I want to LIVE!!

I want to LOVE

---

[36] Johnny Depp's character in the movie "The Professor".

I want to stir up some shit!

Yes, I might not change the world all on my own, but I know I want to keep on trying. When my children, grandchildren and great-grandchildren ask: "What were you doing when these things were happening?" I want to at least be able to say: "I tried."

I'm prepared for the attacks from those ensconced in the masculine world that patriarchy has created over centuries.

It's never wise to mess with a post-menopausal woman like me.

With my body full of scars, I will pick up my sword and – with apologies to P!nk – spit in the wind and enter into battle while shouting loudly:

"I AM HERE!"[37]

---

[37] P!nk: "I am Here" and "All I know so far".

Postscript

I was back at the gynaecologist for a check-up. It was 366 days since my world started to spin differently on its axis. 366 days of painful healing. 366 days of discovery.

The physical healing was tiring and painful, but nothing compared to the exhaustion and agony of the emotional journey. I had gone to the deepest, darkest corners of my psyche and faced what scared me most.

Sitting in the waiting room amongst women bulging with the imminent arrival of new life, I wondered: "Am I done?"

I knew the answer was no – on more than one level.

I had hoped that after a hard year of introspection I would not only feel physically well again, but also have a sense of inner calm and peace.

I didn't. Quite the opposite.

Physically I had healed. I was strong – possibly stronger than I had ever been. My inner world was a different story.

On my return from my two-month journey, I felt unsettled. There was none of the usual comfort of being back in my own bed, or the joy of rediscovering my familiar neighbourhood and city.

There was just a deep restlessness.

I struggled to understand what was going on.

In the hope of forcing my soul and body to calm down, I meditated. I spoke to friends and therapists. I exercised. Nothing helped. I had hoped that my many fears were laid to rest, but now it felt as if they had returned with a vengeance.

At first, I despaired – wondering if I was fundamentally broken, but over time I have come to accept that soul wounds never completely heal. Like the scars on our skin, they are always there to remind us of the lives we have lived.

Despite the promises of so many self-help books – and I have read hundreds – there is no formula, no quick solution to heal these hurts. All I could do was to remain conscious of them and remind myself that they were part of a life I no longer lived.

So, when my fear of abandonment or my drive to be superwoman inevitably reappear, I will remind myself that they are the wounds of my childhood, wounds that no longer serve me.

I now know that these wounds can't be suppressed or forced away.

Dealing with these injuries requires gentleness and patience, because they are the wild animals of my soul and like any wild animal they are not easily tamed.

Over the last decade I have been on numerous wilderness

hikes amongst the wild animals of Africa. The guides require absolute silence and concentration so that you can stay alert to the camouflaged presence of predators – lions, leopards or big giants like elephants and rhinos.

After a few days, you become more attuned to nature and often your only warning is a sudden sense of unease.

On one of these hikes, I woke up one night. As always, we were sleeping on the ground under the stars with only a small fire to deter predators. I slowly lifted my head and in the soft haze of the moonlight, I saw a white rhino quietly grazing between the sleeping hikers. With bad eyesight but excellent smell, the three-ton animal gently sniffed her way around the bundles in sleeping bags. I was absolutely entranced.

I looked over to where one of the guides was. He was wide awake and signalled to me to stay very quiet. The rhino was majestic and calm, but like all wild animals could instantaneously become deadly when given a fright.

Growing up in Africa, I was taught early on that when encountering animals in the wild, you should stop and respectfully acknowledge their presence. If you run or approach them aggressively, they will almost certainly attack you. So, all you can do is wait, watch and breathe until they eventually turn around and leave – as the rhino did that night.

Since my operation, I have come to understand that the inner wilderness of my soul requires the same approach. The inner animals of fear and anxiety will always be there.

All I can hope for is that I spot them in time, acknowledge their presence, breathe quietly and wait for them to retreat.

The shyness of the soul demands a gentle approach. As brilliant Celtic theologian John O' Donohue writes in his book *Anam Cara*, "the neon light (of modern consciousness) is too direct to befriend the shadowed world of the soul." If I went in too fast or aggressively, my inner fears would retaliate and attack.

I have accepted that in order to read the signs and spot their appearances in time, I need to have silence in my life. Just as in the wild, I am not able to register the sense of unease if I am surrounded by constant chatter and noise.

That might mean taking time out and "disappearing" from my life, as I did with my two- month walkabout, or perhaps taking one day a week off. At a minimum I know that I have to spend some time every day checking in with my inner wilderness to see which animals are showing up in my soul world at that moment.

On my desk I have a quote from actress Michaela Cole's Emmy acceptance speech. She said: "Do not be afraid to disappear. From it. From us. For a while. And see what comes to you in the silence."

I like that. I know that this is what my, and perhaps all our souls, need to survive.

I have also had to face the fact that we can never get back to who we were before.

A while ago, my son thought it would be hilarious to leave a fresh snakeskin under the pillows on my bed. A very poisonous Cape Cobra had crossed his path on a bike ride that morning and afterwards he spotted the freshly shed skin, which he later placed under my pillows. Needless to say, I didn't quite share the joke.

After the initial shock – and fury at my son – I was fascinated by the skin. Like all snakes, this cobra had become too big, and to keep growing, had to burst out of her skin.

No wonder that in mythology snakes are revered as symbols of transformation and healing.

During my divorce and later after Gerry's death, I often remarked that it felt like someone had torn my skin off and that I had to wait for a new one to grow.

With the hysterectomy, the doctors literally tore my skin open in order to remove the tumour. I had to wait for the skin to regrow so that the wound would close. Though today there is only a thin red scar as a reminder of that drastic invasion, my body and mind will never be or feel the way they did before the operation.

When I came back from my two-month journey in Europe and Africa, I opened my cupboard to find some clean clothes. "Whose clothes are these?" I wondered for a split second. I knew that they were mine, but they felt wrong and strange. There was nothing that I felt comfortable putting on anymore.

It was as if I had come to inhabit a new body and soul, because my old life had become too small for the new me. I had, over the previous year, shed my old skin and now – as uncomfortable as it might be – ready or not, it was time to move forward.

I have surrendered to the possibility that I'm not quite ready to settle down again. I have accepted that the restlessness might be a subconscious push to keep on searching – to continue growing, to keep on shedding skin.

To live a conscious and fulfilling life, I have to keep looking at myself with curiosity. I have to keep asking questions and sit with deeply uncomfortable answers, because once this growth process stops, it will be a sign of physical and/or emotional death.

Back at the gynaecologist, I looked at the pregnant women around me. I too was entering a new stage of my life. It was 32 years to the day since the birth of my first child. It had been exactly two years since my last period and one year since the hysterectomy.

I would never be able to give birth to another human being again, but soon, my daughter would give birth to my first grandchild.

So, the cycle of life continues, and I will enter a new phase of mothering,

But: I am also determined to find my own way of "giving birth" again. What form that will take, I am not yet sure.

What I do know is that I am not done. Like millions of older women all over the world, I will claim my place in the world. I will demand to be seen and to be heard and I will insist that we are central to making this world a better place.

The discovery of the tumour was a watershed moment in my life. After eyeballing death, I knew that I had to figure out what I wanted to do with the rest of my life. To do that, I had to investigate who I was, who I wanted to be and why I was on this earth.

Today, I know for certain that I am someone who loves deeply. I have a soft open heart, but I become a fearless warrior in the face of injustice. I also know that despite my deep need for silence and retreat, I was born to be a voice, to talk about things we often don't dare talk about... like hysterectomies.

For all of this I make no apology.

I did not want to have a hysterectomy – ever – but I now know it inspired me to embark on a journey toward true freedom. The process of wintering has been long and hard, but now the ice is thawing, and spring is coming.

So, it wasn't a waste after all.

It is often easier to stay in winter,
Burrowed down in hibernation nests, away from the
glare of the sun.
But we are brave and a new world awaits us,
Gleaming and green, alive with the beat of wings.

We who have wintered have learned some things.
We sing it out like birds.
We let our voices fill the air.

From "Wintering" by Katherine May

<u>Thank You</u>

So many people helped me to recover and held my hand during the difficult journey of self-discovery:

My daughter, Wilmé, selflessly cared for me for weeks. She was and remains my rock and without her I would not have managed. My son, Wian, made me laugh during his frequent check-ins from abroad. Following the surgery, it was painful, but so uplifting.

Prof. Hennie Botha not only expertly performed the surgery but was a comforting and compassionate presence during the scariest and darkest moments of my life.

Inge Croy and Marty van Schalkwyk journeyed with me during the months of rehab and knew when to push and when to comfort me.

As she has done so often during the last 30 years, Nomajoni Makoena stepped in when the crisis came and with her gentle, quiet presence made life so much easier.

Wendy Scurr and Abraham le Roux listened and helped me to get to grips with the trauma and psychological challenges after the operation.

Malcolm Nicholls and Erwann Fabre two extraordinary healers who listened and walked with me.

Brid Walls and Elaine Desmond have walked with me

through some of the darkest moments of my life the last two decades and were there again.

From all the corners of the world the extraordinary women from the Women's Circle held and comforted me during our monthly sessions.

The people of Aravon writers' retreat provided a space for me to write. The two weeks at this magical place in Wales, was some of the best times of my life.

My dear friend Peter Storey took on the difficult task of editing the book. Most importantly he cheered me on when I doubted myself.

Paul Feldstein believed in this book – this time not only as an agent, but also publisher. We have walked a long road together over the years and it has been a real joy to work together again.

Without all of you this book would not have been written.

Thank you so much.

*****

Join Melanie for "Never waste a good hysterectomy: the podcast" where we discuss all issues hysterectomy related. Scan the QR code for link.

Available on Apple podcast, Spotify, Google podcast and all other major platforms

Printed in Great Britain
by Amazon

37332632R00138